THE GARL

Dr Reg Saynor MSc, PhD, C. Chem, FRSC and FIMLS is a consultant Lipidologist and formerly Laboratory Director of the Cardiothoracic Unit, Northern General Hospital, Sheffield. He was first involved in garlic and onion research nearly thirty years ago, particularly relating to the garlic effect in preventing heart disease and he and his colleagues presented their latest findings in 1994.

Dr Reg Saynor's other main research into fish oil was reported in *The Eskimo Diet* of which he was the co-author.

He has given interviews on radio and television, held seminars and had many articles published throughout the United States, Europe, Canada and Scandinavia.

Also by Dr Reg Saynor (with Frank Ryan)

The Eskimo Diet

THE GARLIC EFFECT

Dr Reg Saynor

Hodder & Stoughton

First published in Great Britain in 1995 by Hodder & Stoughton
A division of Hodder Headline PLC

10 9 8 7 6 5 4 3 2 1

British Library Cataloguing in Publication Data
Saynor, Reg
Garlic Effect
I. Title
615.324324

ISBN 0 340 64031 6

Printed and bound in Great Britain by
Cox & Wyman Ltd, Reading for
Hodder and Stoughton
A Division of Hodder Headline PLC
338 Euston Road
London NW1 3BH

ACKNOWLEDGEMENTS

First and foremost I must thank my wife, Margaret, for her help and advice and for assisting with the compilation and testing of the recipes. My sincere thanks must also go to Dr Julian Gunn, Mr Tim Gillott and other colleagues at the Cardiothoracic Unit, Northern General Hospital, Sheffield. I would like to acknowledge the help of Mr David Roser of the Garlic Research Bureau for imparting some of his wide knowledge of garlic. I must not forget Ms Rowena Webb, Ms Dawn Bates, Ms Rachel Bond, Ms Esther Jagger and other friends at the publishers, for their invaluable help and guidance.

Finally, I wish to acknowledge the help of the late Professor Walter Bartley, whose help in opening those early doors made all my research possible.

Author's Note

This book is intended as a guide to people who want to improve and maintain their health. The remedies it describes are not intended to replace conventional medical treatment. If you are concerned in any way about your health, you should seek medical advice. Do not stop taking any prescribed medication without first consulting your doctor.

CONTENTS

Acknowledgements   v
Introduction   ix

PART 1: ALL ABOUT GARLIC AND HEALTH   1

1 Know Your Onions   **3**
Garlic in History, Myth and Legend   3
The Chemistry and Botany of the Onion Family   15

2 Keep Your Life Blood Flowing with Garlic   **21**
Cholesterol and the Blood Fats   21
The Heart and Circulation   37
Coronary Thrombosis   46
High Blood Pressure   55

3 On the Brink of New Discoveries   **61**
A Natural Antibiotic   61
Cancer Prevention   65
Garlic Against Free Radicals   70
Diabetes   73

4 Garlic Remedies for Everyday Ailments   **75**
Colds and Flu   75
Sinusitis   76
Sore Throat and Coughs   76

Earache   76
Spots and Boils   77
Acne   77
Warts and Veruccas   78
Athlete's Foot   78
Garlic as a Mosquito Repellent   79
Parasites and Intestinal Worms   79
Sprains   79
Arthritis   80
Indigestion and Diarrhoea   80
Piles and Varicose Veins   80
Chilblains   81
Male Impotence   81

5 Balancing Your Diet with Garlic   83
The Biochemistry of our Bodies   84
The Western Diet and Its Faults   90
How to Take Your Daily Garlic   98

PART 2: RECIPES   101

Soups, Starters and Snacks   105
Main Meals: Poultry   121
Main Meals: Fish   129
Main Meals: Meat   149
Vegetarian Dishes   163
Accompaniments to Other Dishes   169

Source References   174
Further Reading   175
Useful Addresses   176
Index   177

INTRODUCTION: WHY ANOTHER BOOK ON GARLIC?

Nearly fifty years ago, when I was a young, newly married man, I thought it remarkably courageous of my father-in-law to eat a raw onion as readily as I would eat an apple. Nor was it an occasional onion, but a daily one. It was as though he believed an onion a day would keep the doctor away; in his case, it did, despite a very demanding and stressful job. Before departing for work each morning, his breakfast consisted of two or three slices of bread spread with beef or pork dripping, accompanied by a cup of tea. Lunch was usually a piece of hard cheese and a whole raw onion, followed by grapefruit. In all the time I new him, from 1948 until his death in 1989, well into his nineties, he never suffered from a cold or flu.

I often mentioned my father-in-law's dietary habits to my medical colleagues. In the early days, this produced some rather unbelieving looks and remarks – folk remedies were hardly fashionable then among the highly trained members of the medical profession. Some of my colleagues, however, were prepared to listen to me.

I suppose if I was writing a novel I would go on to say that I rushed into the laboratory and started research into onions and garlic, published the results and, in due course, received a Nobel Prize for Medicine. Nothing could be further from the truth, and it was not until the late 1960s that I found an opportunity to test my theory that onion and garlic could help combat coronary heart disease. Since then, many books and articles have been written about the benefits of garlic as a cookery ingredient and, more recently, as an aid to good health.

Garlic possesses many active compounds that give it antibacterial, antibiotic and antioxidant properties. Claims have been made for its efficacy in the treatment of a vast range of ailments and conditions, including heart disease, high blood pressure, arthritis, colds, allergies, intestinal parasites and dysentery.

I chose the present time to add to the literature on garlic because what was hitherto purely anecdotal evidence of its protective effect on the heart and circulation is now acquiring scientific proof. When I started my research on garlic in 1967, I was thought to be somewhat eccentric. But now, nearly thirty years later, the evidence is there – we know it works.

Heart disease is still the commonest cause of death in the United Kingdom and in many other countries in the Western world. In the UK, it accounts for over 150,000 deaths each year. Heart disease is also responsible for many disabilities that prevent the sufferer leading a normal life. Contrary to popular belief, heart disease doesn't affect just one particular social group or sex – it kills people from all walks of life, among them an ever-increasing number of women.

We must all take responsibility for our own health. In order to prevent the accumulation of cholesterol and the formation of blood clots, which ultimately lead to heart attacks and to blocked blood vessels elsewhere in the body, we need to adopt a common-sense approach and tackle a number of habits and beliefs that are doing us no good. Regular exercise, stopping smoking, eating a sensible diet – the benefits of these are all common knowledge, and I shall not elaborate on them. But now we have a new weapon in the armoury – the regular consumption of garlic and onion.

Garlic and onion are both members of the genus *Allium* and have similar effects on our health, although garlic, weight for weight, is much more potent than onion. In Britain and the USA, the odour of garlic on people's breath is considered to be offensive. (Later in this book, I describe ways of counteracting it.) Interestingly, both these countries still have one of the highest levels of coronary heart disease in the world. Mild social unacceptability would seem to be a small price to pay for improving the quality and length of one's life. The inhabitants of the Mediterranean countries suffer no such qualms. There, garlic has been grown and consumed for thousands of years, and it may be no coincidence that heart disease is much less prevalent.

But, if we cannot overcome our dislike of 'garlic breath', there is good news. From the health viewpoint, the most efficient form of garlic is the capsule, which does not smell – so it is possible to eat your cake and have it, too!

I have talked specifically about heart and circulatory diseases because, in this context, I have the support of scientific findings. However, there is also evidence, both anecdotal and scientific, to lead us to believe that garlic is extremely helpful in allaying a number of other medical conditions, both minor and major. The evidence is presented in this book, together with my conclusions.

In the coming decades, the humble garlic bulb and, to a lesser degree, its relatives the onion and the leek, could prove to be the medical salvation of the Western world.

Dr Reg Saynor

Part 1: All about Garlic and Health

1

KNOW YOUR ONIONS

Garlic in History, Myth and Legend

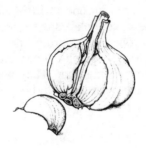

'...a remedy for all diseases and hurts. It provokes urine, and women's courses, helps the biting of mad dogs and other venomous creatures, kills worms in children, cuts and voids tough phlegm, purges the head, helps the lethargy, it is a good preservative against and a remedy for any plague, sore or foul ulcers...'

Nicholas Culpeper, *Complete Herbal*, 1653

The history of the role of garlic in human health is fascinating. Culpeper, although he was writing nearly 350 years ago, was a relative newcomer to the subject. More than a thousand years ago, garlic was used in India for the treatment of diseases of the heart and circulation And, going back several thousand years, earlier civilisations, too, employed garlic for medicinal purposes.

ANCIENT EGYPT

A number of Ancient Egyptian writings and carvings describe the health-giving properties of garlic. Among the extraordinary collection of grave foods buried with the boy-king Tutankhamun were several garlic bulbs – probably to protect him on his journey to the afterlife. Images of garlic bulbs have also been found at a 5,000-year-old burial ground in El Mahasana, but it is not recorded whether these were placed there because of their medicinal or culinary properties. During the Third and Fourth Dynasties (2800-2100 BC) onions, too, were regularly used as offerings, and to decorate the altar. They were buried with the dead, and remains have been found in body cavities such as the thorax and pelvis.

An Essential for the Pyramid Builders

We think of industrial strikes as a comparatively recent phenomenon. In fact, the construction of the Great Pyramid of Cheops at Giza was delayed because of industrial action. When the workers' precious supply of garlic was stopped, they downed tools and refused to continue. Not only did garlic add flavour to their food but, they maintained, it gave them the strength to do their work and it protected them from illness. Let's look at some of the evidence.

First, garlic is known to deter biting insects which, in the Middle East, carry a number of potentially fatal diseases.

Garlic Takes Care of the Nippers
A heart surgeon colleague and his two children had always suffered from the attentions of voracious local mosquitoes on their regular holidays in Tuscany. However, his wife heard that taking one garlic capsule a day (see page 97) might help. One of the children quite enjoyed taking the capsules, and continued them throughout the year, but his brother refused to do so. The next year on holiday in Italy, the regular garlic-taker was completely free from mosquito bites, while his brother received their undivided attention.

Secondly, the Ancient Egyptians had great problems with mouth abscesses. This was because the abundant grain from the fertile land bordering the Nile was ground into flour between two gigantic stones. The flour therefore contained a quantity of finely ground stone, which damaged the Egyptians' teeth. As their teeth slowly wore down, gum abscesses formed. The only treatment they knew of was the regular application of crushed garlic . When this was applied to the teeth and gums, it appeared to have healing properties, as well as an ability to soothe the quite severe pain.

Instinct and Experience

Thirty-five centuries ago, in an Ancient Egyptian manuscript known nowadays as the Codex Ebers, garlic was cited as being useful in the treatment of heart disease, tumours, worms, bites and many other ailments. The Egyptians were basing their knowledge on generations of experience; these days we have the scientific proof. My colleagues and I have demonstrated that garlic can produce significant and beneficial changes in cholesterol and triglyceride, while other researchers have shown that garlic can prevent the formation of clogging materials in the arteries. So, the Egyptians got it right.

THE CHINESE CONNECTION

Although less well documented than the history of garlic in Ancient Egypt, the Chinese interest in the herb goes back much further. When garlic was first grown is not recorded, but it is thought that its cultivation for both culinary and medicinal purposes began, several thousands of years ago, on the lower slopes of the Tien Shan or 'Heavenly Mountains', a range separating China and what was the eastern boundary with the USSR. This area boasted fertile and mineral-rich soil, and had an abundant water supply from the mountains.

China was a great trading nation, and garlic probably spread to the Middle East and Europe via the camel caravans that plied the Silk Road with their burdens of cloth, tea and spices.

Longevity seems to have been one of the main reasons why the ancient Chinese used garlic. They strongly believed that its regular inclusion in their diet would lead to a long and healthy life. One ancient writer went so far as to suggest that if, when a person reached the age of fifty, he ate garlic for fifty days, he would live a further fifty years.

China's Terracotta Army

The Terracotta Army, a collection of thousands of life-size military clay figures, was excavated some time ago in China. Buried alongside the figures were clay models of garlic bulbs, suggesting that garlic was a regular ingredient in the military diet. Maybe garlic was also used by the warriors to protect them during their travels, and during their final journey to the next world.

Fred and His Dog

This is a true story told to me by a colleague. A patient of his called Fred developed severe heart problems in his early sixties. He was warned to live one day at a time and to take things easy – the prognosis was not good. Fred had heard that garlic had been recommended for many years as a protection against heart disease, so he decided to give it a try; it could do no harm, and it was just possible it could help him. Fresh garlic was not part of his usual menu – it does not go well with fish and chips or bacon and egg – so he purchased a pack of one-a-day garlic oil capsules. Now a very fit eighty-five, Fred still takes these capsules regularly.

Incidentally, Fred's dog also received one garlic oil capsule daily, and lived to the venerable age of eighteen.

OTHER MIDDLE EASTERN CULTURES

Flight from Egypt

The Bible contains a reference to garlic in the Book of Numbers (chapter 11, verse 5), which describes the Israelites' flight from Egypt. The Israelites had become accustomed to taking garlic and onion whilst in captivity, and were unhappy to be deprived of them throughout their escape.

The Phoenicians

A nation of international traders and sailors, the Phoenicians came from what is now Lebanon and regularly voyaged to a

number of European countries. During their travels they are likely to have carried garlic as a food flavouring and, perhaps more
importantly, as a remedy for many ailments. This is possibly
how use of the herb spread to Spain, France and other parts of
Europe. It may be that, when the Phoenicians traded with the
people of Cornwall, they introduced garlic to Britain. There is
certainly evidence that the Phoenicians visited Cornwall to buy
the locally mixed tin.

THE GREEKS HAD A WORD FOR IT

Actually, the Greeks had two words for garlic: 'sacred moly' was
how Homer described it in the *Iliad*, claiming magical properties
for the herb. The athletes of Ancient Greece regarded it as an
essential part of their diet when preparing for competitions. The
Greeks also regarded garlic as an aphrodisiac, which may well be
true. Research has shown that, when garlic or onions are consumed, the blood clots less readily and flows more vigorously.
This could account for the increased stamina felt by the field
athletes, and could also improve the blood supply to the penis,
thereby increasing sexual stamina (see Chapter 4).

The Roots of Modern Medical Science

When a doctor qualifies, before being allowed to practise he or
she must take the Hippocratic Oath – an undertaking to treat
each patient to the best of his or her ability, and to uphold the
patient's privacy. The Greek physician Hippocrates, by his scientific, as opposed to mythical, explanations of diseases and
their cures, is regarded as the founder of modern medicine.

The Greek physicians prescribed garlic extensively for many
ailments of the respiratory tract, including bronchitis and pneumonia. In the hands of Hippocrates himself, it became an even
more powerful weapon in the doctor's armoury.

Gangrene is an infection caused by *Clostridium welchii*, a bacterium which spreads rapidly and causes the infected tissues to die. It often occurs when the tissues have been deprived of some of their oxygen and nutrients by the destruction or narrowing of the blood vessels. Even today it is an extremely dangerous condition which, if not treated promptly, can result in amputations and even death. Nevertheless, in around 430 BC, Hippocrates claimed to have treated gangrene with garlic.

The use of garlic as an antibiotic is dealt with more extensively in Chapter 3.

GARLIC IN ROMAN TIMES

Although Rome was a powerful military and political force, much of its cultural, medical and scientific knowledge came from its neighbours the Greeks, who were frequently the (better-educated) slaves of Romans. Galen, a Greek, was physician to the Emperor Marcus Aurelius, and lectured extensively in Rome on herbal medicine. It was through the Greeks that the benefits of garlic as both food and medicine were accepted into the Roman way of life.

The Roman writer Columella seems to have coined the term *unionem*, the precursor of our English world 'onion', in AD 42. It is reported that leeks were used by the Emperor Nero to help him speak more clearly by removing mucus from his throat.

Excavations also tell us a lot about what the Romans ate. The eruption of the volcano Vesuvius in AD 79 destroyed the town of Pompeii; carbonised samples of garlic and onion were subsequently found in digs here and at Herculaneum, which was destroyed at the same time.

A Roman Cure for Boils

Garlic was in common use in Roman times as an effective cure for abscesses and boils. The garlic was dried and ground, and the resulting powder mixed with goose grease and hot ashes before being applied to the affected area. Some writers contend that the ashes were used to open up the boil, so as to allow the garlic to penetrate and destroy the germs. Garlic is a powerful antibacterial agent, so this aspect of their hypothesis is quite credible. The suggested role of the ashes, however, is less plausible – it would have been quicker and more effective to lance the boil with a knife.

Roman Cleanliness – and the Lack of it

The Romans were great engineers; they were renowned for their roads, usually built in a straight line regardless of the difficulty of the terrain. They also built great aqueducts for supplying water, and were famous for their public baths. However, cleanliness was the privilege of the upper classes; the vast majority of the population lived in abject poverty and squalor and was constantly exposed to infection. Knowledge of safe food preparation and preservation was virtually non-existent, and many infections could have been caught through eating contaminated food, as well as through poor personal hygiene.

It was perhaps fortunate, therefore, that most of the population ate garlic which, with its known antibacterial effect, could provide some protection against stomach upsets (see Chapter 3). And, of course, healers would have been able to make effective remedies from garlic and onion.

A Greek in Britain with the Romans

Since the Romans owed so much of their culture and medicine to the Greeks, it comes as no surprise to find that the surgeon general to Julius Caesar's army in 55 and 54 BC was Dioscorides, a Greek physician. He used garlic extensively in the treatment of health problems among the Roman legions invading Britain. Through Dioscorides' guidance, the troops regularly chewed garlic to protect themselves against lung and respiratory diseases, and also to keep their strength up. Stamina was all-important when the legions were on the march, covering distances of thirty miles or more in a single day. The damp climate would have been a valuable ally to the Ancient Britons, for the Romans found our weather pretty inhospitable. Garlic helped them to keep many debilitating illnesses at bay. As time went on, the medicinal use of garlic was taken up by the natives, too.

If the Phoenicians did not bring it earlier, this is probably how garlic was introduced to Britain. It seems very likely that it subsequently played a large part in treating diseases such as cholera, leprosy and typhus. It could help to reduce fevers, destroy the organisms in respiratory diseases, and kill the bacteria causing diarrhoea, which up to that time must have affected most of the population for most of the time.

GARLIC IN MEDIEVAL TIMES AND LATER

During the Middle Ages garlic had become an important part of the European diet and was a valuable item of trade. Two famous sixteenth-century herbal practitioners, Paracelsus and Lonicerus, recognised its effectiveness as an antitoxic agent. Lonicerus also described its effectiveness against intestinal worms, a condition which must have affected large numbers of the population in the Middle Ages. A German herbal called the *Neue Kreuterbuch*, published in 1626, recommended garlic for chills, flatulence, colic and worms.

Shakespeare mentions the pungency of garlic on a number of occasions in his plays. In *Measure for Measure* (Act III, Scene II), Lucio criticises the Duke who, he says, '...would mouth with a beggar though she smelt brown bread and garlic'. In *A Midsummer Night's Dream* (Act IV, Scene II), Bottom tells his fellow actors to eat neither garlic nor onion '...for we are to utter sweet breath'.

Henry IV of France (1566-93) was described in a contemporary document as 'chewing garlic and having breath that would fell an ox at twenty paces'. Later, in 1607, Sir John Harrington wrote in *The English Doctor*:

> Sith Garlicke then hath power to save from death,
> Bear with it though it make unsavoury breathe,
> And scorne not Garlicke like some that thinke,
> It only makes men winke and drinke and stinke.

The Plague

The Middle Ages are often remembered for what was probably the most disastrous epidemic in European history, the Black Death. This outbreak of bubonic plague spread slowly across Asia and Europe, reaching England in 1349. The plague struck again in epidemic proportions in 1665. On both occasions it infected and killed millions of people throughout Europe, sometimes wiping out whole towns and villages.

In those days it was usual to burn sulphur in the hope of killing the organism which caused the disease. Although not always particularly effective, it may have been prompted by the habit of eating garlic. The sulphur compounds in garlic are exhaled from the lungs, and the aroma is also exuded by the skin because of the sulphur molecules that collect in it. The plague-carrying fleas would have been deterred from biting those who were regular garlic eaters.

Garlic Breath can be Life-Saving

In Cheshire, in the north of England, there is a house in which, during the Plague of 1665, garlic was stored. All the inhabitants of the house were unaffected by the disease, and it is thought that the strong aroma of garlic was responsible for this fortunate escape from almost certain death.

In France, it was the practice to make criminals enter houses to remove dead plague victims, who were then transported on carts to the plague pits for mass burial. Four thieves who were made to do this but survived the experience, appeared to get their protection from drinking wine vinegar containing crushed garlic. This tipple, known as *vinaigre des quatre voleurs*, or 'Four Thieves' Vinegar', is still made in France.

OUR OWN TIMES

On the Battlefield

Mrs Beeton, in her famous Victorian cookery book, did not consider garlic suitable for regular use in the kitchen. She recommended that its use should be limited to an occasional light wipe round the salad bowl. In fact, the culinary use of garlic in Britain had already all but disappeared by the beginning of the nineteenth century.

During the First World War, however, garlic was used by the Russians as a treatment for gangrene. Crushed garlic was placed on a dressing improvised from sphagnum moss and applied directly to the wound. It was so effective that during the Second World War garlic was known as 'Russian penicillin'.

In the Jungle

Between 1913 and 1965, the famous medical missionary Dr Albert Schweitzer had a clinic and hospital at the jungle village of Lamberene in Gabon in West Africa. Garlic was his main source of antibacterial treatment, and he claims to have had success in treating long-standing dysentery.

RELIGION AND MYTH

It is well known that garlic is reputed to have the power to repel vampires and evil spirits but, of course, there is no hard evidence! However, garlic and onions have certainly been used in religious ceremonies over hundreds of years. When Satan emerged from the Garden of Eden after Adam's downfall, onions grew from the soil of his right footprint and garlic from that of his left.

But, whatever the truth about claimed magical powers in former times, today's scientific proof makes garlic a piece of modern magic for thousands of sufferers from heart disease.

The Chemistry and Botany of the Onion Family

The botanical name for garlic is *Allium sativum* and it belongs to a large plant family which also includes onions, leeks, chives and shallots. Eating more of any of these plants is a good, healthy decision, but garlic is undoubtedly the most effective of them. It can also be obtained in carefully measured quantities in capsule form.

GROWING GARLIC

Garlic is not a difficult plant to cultivate in the garden, even in the UK and as far north as Sheffield. It is also an excellent organic deterrent against garden pests – any plants growing alongside garlic will not be attacked. Plant individual cloves in October, just as you would a daffodil or tulip bulb. Plant them in a well-drained soil about six inches (15cm) apart, leaving the tips just protruding through the surface of the soil. Do not over-tend or over-water, taking care not to damage the shallow roots. They will be ready to harvest in July or August when the tops are beginning to die down.

WHAT DOES GARLIC CONTAIN?

Numerous investigations have been carried out into the volatile compounds and flavour of garlic and onion. However, until recently there have been few studies into the complete chemical composition of garlic. Despite periods of unfashionability, garlic has long been considered important for its culinary and medicinal uses. But, unlike many vegetables, it has not usually been considered an important source of nutrients. However, garlic has now been shown to contain many of the minerals vital to human health, in particular selenium, which, together with vitamins C and E, makes up part of the body's antioxidant system (see Chapter 3).

Allicin, the 'Miracle Molecule'

It has been suggested that the principal active component of garlic is a substance called allicin, and that the products of its breakdown are sulphides. An uncut clove of garlic or onion has no characteristic strong odour; this only develops when it is broken into. When the cells that make up the garlic clove are cut or damaged, they release two substances: allin and allinase. The latter is an enzyme which combines with the allin to produce allicin, and hence the familiar pungent smell.

Allicin starts to degrade from the moment it is produced, but the speed of this reaction depends on temperature. A few days after it has been produced, allicin can still be detected if the garlic is kept refrigerated, but at room temperature it rapidly breaks down into other products. For some time now, there have been claims that allicin is the 'magic ingredient' in garlic – the constituent which is medically beneficial. But this claim is now virtually disproved. It is likely that the benefit comes from the by-products of the breakdown of allicin, the sulphides.

If you are interested in reading more about allicin, I recommend *Garlic for Health* by David Roser, Director of the Garlic Research Bureau, who calls it the 'miracle molecule'.

The Sulphide Story

Dr Philip Barlow and his colleagues at the University of Humberside have been engaged for a number of years in research on the wide range of available garlic products, and have published a number of excellent scientific papers on the subject. They have looked into claims that dried garlic is the best source of allicin when compared with garlic oil, and found that few, if any, of the products tested (dried garlic powder and garlic oil used in capsules) contained any allicin. They concluded that the activity of garlic as a means of lowering the cholesterol in the blood (see Chapter 2) is linked to the sulphide content.

As allicin breaks down it takes up oxygen from the surrounding air which assists its conversion into sulphur-rich chemicals. There are over seventy of these sulphides, and most of these remain stable − in other words, their chemical form does not change. The fact that there are so many stable sulphides may account for the wide range of illnesses which respond to garlic treatment, because each sulphide reacts in a different way to each disease.

In my early research into the effects of onions on the blood fats of patients with heart disease, I found that the benefits were the same whether the onion was eaten raw, boiled, or fried in vegetable oil. The same seems to hold true for garlic, which strongly suggests that allicin, which is destroyed by heating, is not in itself responsible for garlic's benefits.

But let's go back and look at what happens when we eat raw garlic. Earlier, it was explained that, when garlic is crushed or cut, allicin is released together with its characteristic odour. Exactly the same process applies when garlic is chewed, and the allicin is released into the mouth. Since allicin rapidly breaks down when left at room temperature of around 20°C, when garlic is chewed at the higher temperature inside the mouth the process of breakdown is even faster.

Then, when the garlic is swallowed, it passes into the stomach where it is attacked by hydrochloric acid as digestion starts. The stomach empties its contents into the duodenum, where digestive enzymes act further on the garlic. It is only after the next step, when it moves into the intestine, that absorption into the bloodstream finally takes place. This seems to be pretty conclusive evidence that, if allicin is so sensitive to rises in temperature, it will have been converted into sulphides long before it reaches the point at which it is absorbed into the blood. In fact, it is unlikely that allicin gets beyond the initial chewing process.

Essential Oil of Garlic

Further proof that allicin is not itself the active agent in garlic can be found in the preparation of garlic oil by a process known as steam distillation. In this process, crushed garlic is treated to a high-temperature bath in steam. The oil is leached from the garlic and carried with the steam to a condenser, where the temperature is low enough to change the steam back into water. As oil and water do not mix, the garlic oil floats on the water's surface and can be removed.

The process takes some time, which, combined with the heat to which the oil is subjected, breaks down any allicin present so that only sulphides remain.

Researchers now believe that any action achieved by garlic comes from the components in its oil, and not from the water-based molecules. This was put to the test by boiling garlic in water and testing the activity of both the boiled garlic and the water in which it had been boiled. The result would appear to be conclusive – the garlic was still active, but no activity remained in the water.

Good News from a Japanese Laboratory

Platelets are cellular particles in the blood which release a substance which causes the blood to clot when a vessel is damaged. Chapter 2 describes more about the vital part played by the platelets in clotting and how, paradoxically, they can also contribute to the clogging of vital coronary arteries. New findings now appear to show that garlic can be very useful in helping to keep these vessels clear.

In Japan, a group of researchers have synthetically produced one of the sulphide compounds which appear as a result of the breakdown of allicin. This compound is called *methyl allyl trisulphide* (MATS), and has been thoroughly tested in clinical trials. MATS would seem to be very effective in reducing the platelets' clotting capability and helping to keep the blood flowing freely through the coronary arteries. To benefit from MATS, all you need to do is chew a garlic clove or two daily, or take a Hofel's Cardiomax garlic oil capsule a day (see page 98).

And now let's take a fuller look at what garlic can do for your heart and circulation.

2

KEEP YOUR LIFE BLOOD FLOWING WITH GARLIC

Cholesterol and the Blood Fats

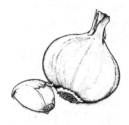

About one in three men and one in four women will suffer a heart-related disease before reaching the age of retirement. A few years ago, women were considered to have a much lower risk of heart attack than men. But times change, and the figures for women are now nearly as high as those for men.

THE WESTERN DIET AND HOW WE COPE WITH IT

Perhaps the most important risk factor in the majority of Western countries is our consumption of food with a high content of saturated fats (see pages 86-89 for definitions of saturated and unsaturated fats, polyunsaturates and monounsaturates).

Some researchers and writers believe that eating a diet rich in saturated fats leads inevitably to cardiovascular disease, but this is not an opinion to which I subscribe. Many people survive into their eighties and nineties on a diet which would lead others to heart surgery in their forties and fifties. However, these lucky people are in the minority, and are often described as 'the survivors' by eminent members of the scientific and medical establishment.

I do not think that this trait of long life in the face of all odds is just a matter of chance, but rather an indication that their bodies deal with saturated fat differently from those of the majority of us. It may be that these fortunate people also regularly eat quantities of garlic and onion and other heart-beneficial foods, such as oily fish (see my earlier book, *The Eskimo Diet*). More fundamentally, their blood fat pattern may be influenced by their consumption of such foods.

But first, I want to explain some of the processes that occur in our bodies.

CHOLESTEROL

Whenever the word cholesterol is mentioned nowadays, most people shrink in horror as if they are preparing to be struck down by some loathsome, oily substance. Nothing could be further from the truth. In fact, cholesterol is an essential component of our body chemistry, and without it we just would not exist.

Cholesterol helps maintain our body cells and initiates the production of bile acids. These acids process fat in our intestines so that it can be absorbed into the bloodstream. Cholesterol is also essential for the production of the sex hormones and, therefore, has a vital role to play in reproduction.

So, it is not nature which has got it wrong – we have. Nature has provided a system that produces sufficient cholesterol for the body's normal requirements. What we have done is to overload that finely tuned mechanism with extra cholesterol taken in from our fatty diet. Dairy products and eggs, and too much red meat and fried food (especially fast food, such as hamburger and chips), all help to increase our intake of saturated fats.

The Vegetable Fallacy

Most people consider that frying in vegetable oil instead of lard or dripping is the healthy option. Indeed, it is – but not always. One fry-up in oil is probably not particularly harmful, but to use the oil more than once or twice is asking for trouble. When unsaturated vegetable oil is heated to a temperature of 190°C and freshly cut chips are added, the chemical reaction that takes place is very similar to the process used by the manufacturers of hard saturated fats. The water in the chips combines with the oil at a high temperature and starts to saturate the unsaturated oil which we started with. As time goes on and the oil is used again and again for frying, more and more saturated fats are formed. You can see it is happening because the oil becomes thicker and more cloudy.

So, it is better to use cooking oil once only, and cut down on bought fast foods where you are not in control of the cooking process and where the oil may well have been used several times over. Note also that not all oils are equal – see page 86-89 for details of which are healthy and which are not.

Cholesterol and Coronaries

Thousands of scientific studies and clinical trials have been conducted into the role of cholesterol in coronary artery disease. The vast majority have demonstrated a strong relationship between excessive blood cholesterol levels and heart disease, although a small percentage of studies have shown no link at all. But it is reasonable to conclude that there would seem to be a high risk of heart attack in the majority of the population of the UK who have high blood cholesterol.

High Cholesterol Doesn't Always Kill

To keep the picture in perspective and, to some extent, play Devil's advocate, I must recount a story about a patient of mine. Some years ago, when I was running a cholesterol clinic, I was asked by a GP to see an elderly man whose blood cholesterol was 12.7 – more than twice the normal level of 6.0. Since the man was eighty-four, it had probably been at that level for many years.

He looked at his diet very carefully, reduced his fat intake to a sensible level and, over a period of a few weeks, his cholesterol came down to 6.1. He lived happily for several more years, eventually dying from a cause completely unrelated to coronary heart disease.

I must stress that this man was one of life's lucky exceptions. For the majority of people, such a high cholesterol level would have resulted in death many years earlier.

Inherited High Blood Cholesterol

Although the majority of people with raised blood cholesterol can reduce it just by altering their diet, there are some who cannot because they suffer from a condition called *familial hyper cholesterolaemia*. In plain language, this means they have an inherited high blood cholesterol level. One person in 500 of the UK population has this problem, and it usually comes to light when he or she mentions to the doctor that several members of his or her family have died young of heart attacks, or suffered sudden death. The heart attack risk for this group of patients is about eight times that of the rest of the population, and it is important to do something about the condition as soon as possible.

If you think you might be affected you should go to your doctor, who will arrange to take a sample of blood for screening. It will be sent to a hospital or laboratory for testing so that a complete fat profile can be established. The tests should include triglyceride (see page 31) and both HDL and LDL cholesterol (see below), with a calculation of your risk factor based on the ratio of LDL to HDL.

Some chemist's shops offer quick cholesterol testing, or kits for you to do it yourself at home, but I regard these as unreliable and misleading. Many people have come to see me reporting a high cholesterol level which, when tested in a specialist National Health Service laboratory, gives an entirely different picture. One of the reasons for this apparent discrepancy is that there are two types of cholesterol: HDL, which is good, and LDL, which is bad.

HDL Cholesterol – the Protector

HDL stands for high-density lipoprotein, a particle which circulates in the blood and picks up excess cholesterol from the body tissues, including the coronary arteries. HDL then returns this unwanted cholesterol to the liver, where it can be either recycled or excreted.

The liver is the organ responsible for the production of cholesterol and the other blood fats. When we talk about a person's HDL cholesterol level, we are referring to the amount of cholesterol being *removed* from the tissues. A high HDL level, therefore, reflects the efficiency of the substance's scavenging function.

Professional Testing Reveals Hidden Risks
One of my patients went to a chemist's shop and had his blood cholesterol measured. The result was an acceptable 5.9. When he came to my laboratory, we found that his cholesterol was near enough to what

> the shop had found. However, we also discovered something that the original test hadn't – his 'protective' HDL cholesterol was only 0.65. This put the man into a high-risk category, and intensive effort was required in order to reduce his risk.
>
> Incidentally, the research undertaken by my colleagues and myself in Sheffield shows that regular consumption of garlic capsules can raise the 'protective' HDL cholesterol level – something not achievable by many of the LDL cholesterol-lowering drugs

A few years ago, an eminent physician in the USA, Dr Castelli, reported a tragic case. A young man in his thirties, apparently fit, was found dead in his bed. At the post-mortem examination, the man's coronary arteries were found to be clogged with atheroma – a build-up of cholesterol and blood fat deposits – which had dramatically reduced the blood flow to his heart. Yet this man had a normal cholesterol level. For this reason, Dr Castelli decided to investigate further.

What he found provided the clearest support for the role of HDL cholesterol in coronary artery disease. Although the man's cholesterol was quite normal, his HDL cholesterol was so low that his ability to remove excess cholesterol from the tissues was greatly impaired, resulting in the clogging of his arteries and subsequent death. Since that time, a great deal of research has been carried out, indicating that the increased risk of heart attacks occurs in those people with a low HDL cholesterol level.

LDL Cholesterol – the Real Killer

LDL, or low-density lipoprotein, is the actual cholesterol-carrying particle. Produced in the liver, it is loaded with cholesterol which it transports around the body, and off-loads into the cells and tissues so that they can function properly (Fig. 1).

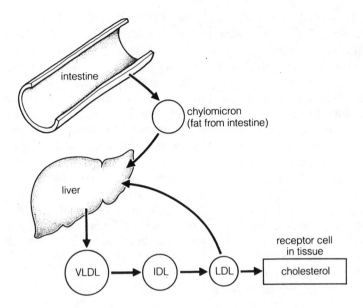

Fig. 1: Production of the LDL (low-density lipoprotein) Particle
Fat from the intestine forms chylomicrons for transport to the liver. The liver incorporates the cholesterol and triglyceride from the chylomicrons into another particle known as VLDL (very low-density lipoprotein). VLDL then gives up its triglyceride to form IDL (intermediate density lipoprotein). From this, LDL, now consisting mostly of cholesterol, is formed. LDL is picked up by the receptors in the cells, and deposits its cholesterol.

It is a complex and wonderful system. The inner lining of the arteries, as well as other tissues, contain special receptor sites for cholesterol, and send chemical messages to the LDL which enable it to carry out accurate deliveries. The problems are caused when we interfere with this finely tuned process by eating too much food containing saturated animal fats. As a result, the receptors in our cells are completely overwhelmed and cannot cope with all the cholesterol being produced. The result is the furring up of the arteries, which gradually deteriorate and provoke coronary artery disease.

If you still need convincing about the importance of reducing cholesterol to lower your risk of heart attack, ask your local library to obtain a copy of the November 1994 issue of the *Lancet*, which contains the important paper by the Scandinavian Simvastatin Survival Group. These researchers discovered that when cholesterol is lowered, in this case by a drug, the incidence of heart attack falls dramatically and the risk of having to undergo heart surgery is reduced by 37 per cent. This should stimulate us all to look closely at our blood cholesterol levels and our diet, and to take the necessary action.

It is helpful as part of this action to discover your blood cholesterol level. Ask your GP if you can have this test done, and request what is known as a 'full lipid profile'. The test will only need to be repeated every two or three years because, unless you make significant changes to your diet, the results are unlikely to alter in such a short period. The exceptions are people with inherited high blood cholesterol, who need regular monitoring by their GP or local hospital.

Garlic and Cholesterol – the Breakthrough

In 1977 I attended a medical conference in Cambridge on HDL (good) cholesterol – possibly the very first on the subject. Dr W. Castelli from the USA talked to us about the dangers of low HDL cholesterol. Unfortunately, he was unable, in those days, to suggest any treatment other than a change of diet, which I found did not work very well.

I came back to my laboratory in Sheffield and, with the help of my colleagues, set up a method for measuring HDL cholesterol. This was no simple matter, and it took many months of concentrated effort. During this period, I spoke to Walter Bartley, Professor of Biochemistry at Sheffield University, about my research work with onions. I suggested that allicin was the active, beneficial component in garlic and onion. He quietly destroyed my argument and suggested that it was the sulphur compounds which were responsible for the benefits, because it was not possible for allicin to remain active after it had entered the mouth.

The breakthrough came in 1992 when my colleagues and I researched the effect of Cardiomax garlic oil capsules on a number of hospital patients. Some had suffered heart attacks, others had high blood pressure, and two were diabetics. All had HDL and LDL cholesterol levels which put them at high risk from further heart problems. These patients had been on a cholesterol-lowering diet for some time, and most had been treated with drugs to the same end. But it was all to no avail: their blood test results remained persistently bad.

Before starting to take the garlic oil, the patients gave blood samples once a week for a month so that we had a consistent baseline against which to compare the new samples. After they had each taken one garlic capsule a day for a further month, the results began to improve. In the second month of treatment, the patients were taking two capsules daily and the effects were even better. The following month, the dose went up to three, with dramatic effects on the patients' LDL cholesterol level. It came down by almost 10 per cent, bringing the level within the safe range. At the same time, their HDL cholesterol increased significantly. Nearly a month after stopping the garlic oil the patients' results had still not returned to the pre-garlic levels. All the patients are now taking one capsule a day and we will measure any changes over the future months.

Garlic and the onion family rapidly became a hot topic for scientific investigation worldwide, and there is only space here to mention one or two of the studies.

Some years after I first began to look into the benefits of the onion family for the control of heart disease, Dr Jain and Dr Vyas reported on their research. They found similar changes to mine, but had also fed onion as well as garlic to their patients. Another researcher, Dr Agusti, gave garlic juice to five patients and saw a massive 30 per cent reduction in bad cholesterol levels. Even when the garlic was stopped, it took two months for the cholesterol to return to its pre-garlic level. We had had exactly the same findings in Sheffield.

Yet another study looked at the cholesterol levels in three groups of people. The first group comprised those who had abstained from garlic all their lives for religious reasons. These people had the highest blood cholesterol levels. The second group had a cholesterol level an average 17 per cent lower: they ate only small amounts of garlic. It was the third group, who consumed liberal amounts of garlic, which had the lowest cholesterol levels of all – 25 per cent lower than group one.

A five-year-long World Health Organisation study of 10,000 men in three countries, reported in 1978 on the effectiveness of a drug called *clofibrate* in lowering cholesterol, and of the subsequent effect on the death rate. The conclusions could not have been clearer: for every 1 per cent fall in cholesterol, there was a 2 per cent fall in heart attack risk. In this study, the cholesterol was reduced by 12 per cent, which one would expect to lead to a high reduction in risk.

In India, Professor Bordia compared the cholesterol-lowering effects of *clofibrate* with those of garlic. He found garlic to be much more effective. In the early 1960s, I had been involved in *clofibrate* research. The cholesterol level of patients taking the drug was effectively reduced and, at the time, many of us thought that here lay the answer to our cholesterol problems. Unfortunately, some years later *clofibrate* had to be withdrawn because of undesirable side-effects. No such problem with garlic: in normal amounts, it will not only sort out your cholesterol problems but add spice to your life and diet, too.

Bordia fed cholesterol to rabbits, and duly found an increase in the bad cholesterol and a decrease in the good cholesterol. This was no surprise – every day millions of humans are doing the same thing by including too much saturated fat in their diet. But when the animals were fed essential oil of garlic, these changes were reversed.

Even more impressively, in a control group of rabbits which was not fed garlic oil, the blood vessels showed severe clogging. But in those taking the garlic oil, the arteries were much clearer.

This is excellent news for us humans who daily feed ourselves large quantities of cholesterol-producing fat. If these animal results can be applied to humans, it means that clogging of the arteries will be dramatically slowed and the heart attack rate possibly reduced.

TRIGLYCERIDES

A major source of energy in our diet, triglycerides are derived from both animals and plants and constitute most of the fats in our fatty tissue. They are called upon to provide energy whenever we are deprived of food. Triglycerides are present in the top of the milk, in cream, and in the white fat on meat which can be reconstituted to make delicious but unhealthy dripping. Triglycerides are one of the body's most important sources of energy – weight for weight, they provide more energy than sugar. They can be absorbed directly from the food we eat, or they may be manufactured in the liver and incorporated into the VLDL (see Fig. 1) and, to some extent, the bad (LDL) and good (HDL) particles.

Triglycerides have two main ingredients: glycerol and fatty acids. When represented diagrammatically, a single glycerol molecule has three arms rather like a trident; bonded to each arm is the second component, the fatty acids (Fig. 2). From this combination of three fatty acids with one molecule of glycerol, we get the term triglyceride.

Blood triglyceride levels vary greatly between individuals. Within an hour or so after a meal, the triglyceride concentration in the blood will rise significantly. This contrasts with cholesterol, which appears relatively unaffected after a meal, instead rising gradually over weeks, months and years.

So, where does triglyceride fit into the heart attack story? Some years ago, Dr Hugh Sinclair examined the Eskimos in their natural environment, and found that their cholesterol level

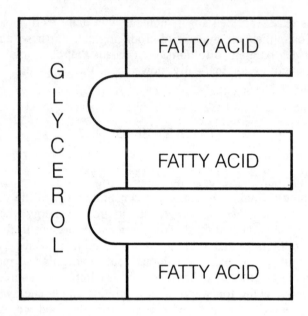

Fig. 2: Diagrammatic representation of a triglyceride molecule

was not far short of that in the UK population, although they had
very few heart attacks the big difference was that the triglycerides of the Eskimos were much lower than those of British
people, which implied that triglycerides played an important part
in heart disease.

The Evidence for Triglycerides as a Risk Factor

In 1993, the *British Medical Journal* published an article by the
Norwegian Dr Stensvold and his colleagues on the role of blood
triglyceride concentrations as a risk factor for coronary heart
disease. Researchers examined 25,058 men and 24,535 women
between the ages of thirty-five and forty-nine. They concluded
that a high, non-fasting blood triglyceride level was a risk factor
for death from coronary heart disease and cardiovascular disease

among women.

Another group, Welin and colleagues, reported in the *European Heart Journal* in 1991 the results of a long-term study which looked at the cholesterol and triglyceride concentrations in two groups of elderly men. One group comprised men who were sixty years old at the start of the study, and the other group sixty-seven. The groups were monitored for seven and eight years respectively. The results were surprising. Both blood triglyceride and cholesterol levels were significant risk factors, but in those men with raised triglycerides, the risk of suffering a heart attack was greater.

Finally, Patsch and colleagues, an eminent group of researchers based in the USA and Austria, found that if the triglyceride level measured at six and eight hours after a fatty meal was high, the risk of coronary heart disease increased.

The evidence is clear.

Fats of Flight

Triglyceride is stored by the body in the adipose tissue – the fat which covers our bodies to a greater or lesser degree. From these stores the body can quickly mobilise the fatty acids required to provide energy at any given moment. I sometimes describe these as the 'fats of flight', and a little story will explain why.

In the days when all we human beings wore was an animal skin and a smudge of woad, and mammoths and sabre-toothed tigers roamed the land, fatty acids were very important. Imagine for a moment early man, out hunting when he hears the roar of a sabre-toothed tiger somewhere behind him. His initial reaction is panic, followed by a desire to run away as quickly as possible. This emotion has the effect of increasing the supply of adrenalin into his bloodstream, which in turn raises his heart, pulse rate and blood pressure in readiness for escape.

But before this can happen, it is necessary for the body to find a source of energy to power the muscles. In fact, the adrenalin also helps to release fatty acids from the body's fat stores. The man can then run until he is out of danger from the tiger, by which time his heart rate, blood pressure and adrenalin will have normalised, the fatty acids having been burned up as energy.

What happens nowadays? Our potential victim is sitting in his office when the phone rings. It's his boss, hauling him over the coals for some dereliction of duty. Immediately, the adrenalin starts to flow, followed by the other effects of blind panic. But, instead of indulging in vigorous 'flight' exercise, our victim sits and lights a cigarette to 'calm his nerves'. All those circulating fatty acids don't get burned off. Instead, they are deposited straight into the body tissues. If this happens continually, our victim could be on the way to an early heart attack.

High Triglycerides Often Means Low HDL

My own research, and that of many others, has shown that people with high triglycerides often have a low HDL (good) cholesterol, and that when the triglyceride is reduced by changes in diet, the HDL increases. This happened to me about twenty years ago when I was found to have a very high blood triglyceride concentration.

Understanding the implications, I immediately switched to a diet which would reduce my triglyceride level – and the effect was almost immediate. Within just a few days my triglyceride had fallen from 4.72 to 1.9 (the normal level is less than 2.0), with a correspondingly effective rise in HDL cholesterol.

The answer to the triglyceride problem is to consume only very small amounts of saturated fat, sugar and alcohol. A glass of wine, particularly red wine, does no real harm – indeed, there is evidence that red wine drunk in moderation can actually protect against heart attacks but difficulties arise when people regularly drink large quantities of beer and spirits. In some cases, it can lead to alarmingly high triglyceride levels. I must emphasise here that this phenomenon does not affect us all, but only a minority whose livers seem to be particularly sensitive to alcohol.

Alcohol and the Triglyceride Switchback

At two o'clock one morning in 1966, a thirty-six-year-old miner was admitted to the hospital at which I work. He had woken with severe chest pain and was sent in with a suspected heart attack.

Because I had expressed an interest in the blood fat pattern of patients with heart problems, the senior registrar asked me to measure this patient's cholesterol and triglyceride levels. In those early days it was not possible to asses HDL cholesterol, and triglyceride tests were in their infancy. Even so, I found that the patient's blood triglyceride was extremely high.

About ten days later it was decided that the patient had not suffered a heart attack at all, but that his pain was probably due to severe indigestion. Before he left, another blood sample was taken and analysed for triglycerides. This time, the result was completely normal. When I talked to the patient, I discovered that on the night he was admitted, he had consumed his customary eight pints of beer. However, the spell in hospital without any access to alcohol except that on the swabs had normalised his blood triglyceride. Sadly, I had little doubt that, within a few days of returning to daily life, his triglycerides would be sky high again.

Triglycerides and Garlic

Our researches at Sheffield, during which we had observed great improvements in HDL cholesterol among patients who were given Cardiomax garlic oil capsules, also disclosed considerably reduced triglyceride levels. In the third month of the treatment, when our patients were up to three capsules a day, their triglyceride fell by a massive 25 per cent!

CHECK YOUR CONTRACEPTION

Certain oral contraceptive pills have a tendency to increase the triglyceride and cholesterol levels in the blood, which is a matter of some concern to women. Your GP or family planning clinic will advise on which pill is most suitable for you, taking into account any blood fat problem you may have. The situation can also be counteracted to some extent by increasing your HDL cholesterol. In general, a sensible diet with plenty of fruit and vegetables, and a reduction in fat and sugar consumption, together with moderate exercise, will help to keep the blood fats in balance. And remember to take your capsules of garlic oil.

The Heart and Circulation

The main purpose of the heart is to pump blood through the arteries to the vital organs of our bodies. Situated behind the sternum or breastbone, the heart is a muscular organ about the size of a man's fist and, although it lies centrally in the upper chest, it has a slight tilt to the left.

Fig. 3 shows the four chambers of the heart – two atria and two ventricles – together with some of the large blood vessels. Remember that you are looking at a mirror image, so right and left appear to be transposed.

A POWERFUL MUSCLE

The human heart continues to beat throughout life at around seventy-two beats a minute when we are at rest. Exercise or stress can cause the number of beats to increase substantially. In the average lifetime, the heart expends sufficient energy to lift a 35,000 ton battleship fourteen feet out of the sea! Every second of every minute of every hour of every day of our lives, the heart circulates oxygen-rich blood to the brain, liver, lungs, kidneys and everywhere else in the body. Without the vital oxygen contained in the blood, the body would rapidly die.

The heart also needs its own, efficient supply of oxygenated blood. It receives this via the coronary arteries. The aorta carries oxygenated blood from the heart, to be distributed, through smaller and smaller arteries, into the organs. As the aorta leaves the heart, it forks into two large arteries. These are the right and left coronary arteries, which supply the heart muscle and pass over the surface of the heart, subdividing into four more, smaller arteries. These arteries split further to form a number of smaller vessels running through the muscles of the heart.

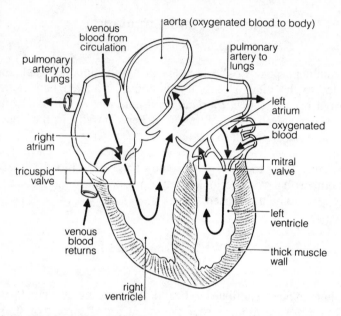

Fig. 3: Chambers of the Heart. The arrows indicate the direction of blood flow.

When we walk or take exercise, our muscles eventually become weary and we feel tired. Obviously, the heart must behave differently, and it is constructed in such a way that it can continue to function without fatigue.

Each side of the heart has two chambers – on the left is the left atrium, which has a thin wall and sits on top of the highly muscular left ventricle, from which it is separated by the mitral valve. The right side of the heart has a similar structure, with the right atrium and right ventricle separated by the tricuspid valve. The function of both valves is to allow blood to flow in one direction only. The tricuspid valve is so called because it consists of three small flaps. The mitral valve gets its name because its shape resembles a bishop's mitre.

The muscle wall of the left ventricle is thicker than that of the right ventricle. This is because the left ventricle has to exert more pressure than the right. The normal heartbeat consists of two sounds; the first sound is that of the contraction of the two atria, which pump blood under low pressure (hence their less muscular wall construction) through the valves into the right and left ventricle.

THE CIRCULATION IN THE HEART

Blood which has given up most of its oxygen during its journey through the body is known as deoxygenated blood. It returns, through the veins, into the right atrium and then to the right ventricle. From here it is pumped into the pulmonary artery to enable it to become oxygenated again on its journey through the lungs. On returning to the heart, the blood passes into the left atrium, and from there through the mitral valve into the left ventricle, where it is pumped at high pressure and leaves the heart through the aorta. This, the largest artery in the body, then distributes oxygenated blood to all the tissues of the body. In order to prevent the blood, which is under high pressure, from flowing backwards at the end of this cycle, there are valves in the pulmonary artery and aorta which snap shut; this is what produces the second sound of the normal heartbeat.

THE HEART'S PACEMAKER

In order to pump the blood, the chambers of the heart need to contract in a particular sequence, for which a sophisticated control mechanism is provided. The heart's own tiny 'pacemaker', known as the sino-atrial node, is located at the top of the heart. It is connected to the chambers through a system of fibres which pass through the walls of the heart and carry electrical signals to the heart muscles. These signals are produced at a frequency to give seventy-two beats a minute at rest. The well-coordinated movement as the heart beats is produced by the chambers of the heart operating in a rigidly controlled sequence in response to the pacemaker's instructions.

WHAT CAUSES A HEART ATTACK?

If the electrical signal from the sino-atrial node to the heart is blocked or upset in any way, the heart cannot function properly, and a heart attack may result. One of the commonest ways in which this can happen is when a clot appears in a coronary artery, thus interfering with the muscle's ability to contract. The individual conducting fibres can then start to fire electrical signals at random, as a result of which the previously coordinated seventy-two beats a minute cannot be achieved, and the heart goes into a state of fibrillation. In other words, it is unable to pump blood and has the appearance of a trembling jelly. Unless this condition is reversed within three minutes, the patient will die because the vital organs, including the brain, will be starved of oxygen and sustain irreversible damage.

Heart Rhythm and Garlic
When somebody has a heart problem, it is often denoted by a change in the rhythm of the heart. When the coronary arteries are blocked, for instance, the rhythm change is called *ventricular tachycardia*. It is dangerous, and has to be corrected quickly. This can be done by using a defibrillator, which applies a strong electric shock to the heart for a very short time, or with drugs.

Recently, I came across a copy of a medical research paper which described the effect of wild garlic (*Allium ursinum*) on ventricular fibrillation. The research workers in this study had induced ventricular fibrillation in two groups of animals, one of which had previously been fed pulverised wild garlic leaves. In the garlic group, the incidence of fibrillation was reduced by an astonishing 30 per cent when compared with the other group.

(For recipes using wild garlic, see pages 105 to 174)

Atheroma and Angina

The lining of the arteries is covered with living cells, and it is around these that the clot starts with the deposition of a porridge-like substance called atheroma. Atheroma consists of fats, cholesterol, and other materials. As the years pass, more and more atheroma builds up, and the orifice, or lumen, through which blood can flow becomes more and more restricted. (See Fig. 4).

Atheroma forms on damaged cells lining the arteries. How do the cells become damaged in the first place? There are a number of reasons. It is now known that the chemicals produced by smoking (more on this topic below) can damage the lining cells, as can some infections. One of the most important factors involved in producing atheroma, however, is a natural protective process instigated by the body itself.

When you cut your finger, after a few minutes, if the wound is not too severe, a clot forms around the cut. This is the result of a complicated process which brings together, in the correct quantities and sequence, a number of blood factors which react with one another to form the clot, and so stop the bleeding. One of the most important components in clotting is the platelet, which gathers in great numbers around the injury on the blood vessel.

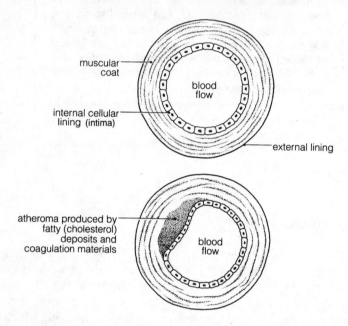

Fig. 4: Cross-section through a normal artery (top) and, below, an artery damaged by atheroma.

This is fine in most circumstances, but platelets also do their clotting, of course, when the inner lining of a coronary artery is damaged. This is considerably less useful, for clotted blood in a damaged coronary artery often means the start of the build-up of atheroma.

If you are lucky enough not to suffer a heart attack through the existence of atheroma, its presence may not be felt until, probably in middle age, a severe pain occurs in the chest and down the arms during normal activity. This pain is known as angina, and occurs when insufficient blood reaches the heart to provide the high level of oxygen required. Often, it happens when other muscles of the body are being exerted, and are therefore competing for the oxygenated blood.

RISK FACTORS FOR HEART DISEASE

Some of these will already have become obvious, while others are dealt with at greater length elsewhere in this book. Here is a résumé of the other major risk factors.

Smoking

It has been known for many years that smoking is responsible for respiratory diseases such as emphysema, chronic bronchitis, lung cancer and so on. But, recently, it has finally been established as a major risk factor in the development of coronary artery disease. Some people think that only cigarettes are to be avoided in this context, but the warning applies to all forms of tobacco, including pipes and cigars.

Over the past two decades or so, the number of men continu-

Bob and His Pipe

A patient who used to visit my lipid clinic had a responsible job, and at the end of a day's work liked to start his evening's relaxation by sitting down to a good cooked dinner. Bob was especially fond of fried foods, such as bacon, sausages and chips. After dinner, he would settle down, switch on the television, light his pipe and puff away contentedly, especially if there was football to watch.

As he got a little older – he was fifty-two when he came to see me – he noticed a strange tingling sensation in his legs when he smoked his pipe in the evening. His wife persuaded him to visit the doctor, who arranged for him to have tests at the local hospital. Bob was found to have peripheral artery disease, which means clogging of the leg arteries, and it became much less noticeable when he finally threw his pipe in the waste bin.

What was happening to Bob was a combination of changes. First, the high saturated fat content of his evening meal had produced a high blood fat level, making his blood thicker and more sluggish, and therefore prone to clot formation. The smoking aggravated this condition, and at the same time stimulated chemical changes which caused the arteries to contract (known as vasoconstriction) and narrow temporarily. This effect, combined with the pre-existing atheroma (present in most of us at Bob's age) restricted the blood flow and caused the odd tingling

ing to smoke has fallen appreciably; but women have been much more resistant to the various anti-smoking campaigns, putting themselves at greater risk. However, hormonal changes contribute to the fact that post-menopausal women now account for over 40 per cent of the death rate from heart disease.

Alcohol

Shakespeare may not have been a heart surgeon, but in *Macbeth* he brilliantly expressed some of the unpleasant effects of over-indulging in alcohol.

Macduff: Was it so late, friend, ere you went to bed, that you do lie so late?

Porter: Faith, sir, we were carousing till the second cock: and drink, sir, is a great provoker of three things.

Macduff: What three things does drink especially provoke?
Porter: Marry, sir, nose-painting, sleep and urine. Lechery, sir, it provokes, and unprovokes: it provokes the desire, but it takes away the performance: Therefore, much drink may be said to be an equivocator with lechery: it makes him, and it mars him; it sets him on, and it takes him of; it persuades him, and disheartens him; makes him stand to, and not stand to: in conclusion, equivocates him in a sleep, and, giving him the lie, leaves him.

Age

Advancing age is a risk factor we can do little about, except to adopt a healthy diet and lifestyle.

Food for Thought

1. A businessperson has a 1 in 3 chance of suffering a heart attack or some other serious illness before retirement age.

2. Only 8 per cent of deaths in the year 1900 were due to heart disease. In 1993, the figure was 35 per cent.

3. Nearly 80 per cent of women and men between the ages of thirty-five and fifty-four are alive five years after their first heart attack.

Coronary Thrombosis

I have already talked a little about the mechanism of clotting and its role in heart attacks. Let's now look at it in a little more detail in relation to coronary artery disease.

Thousands of scientific papers have been written on the subject of clotting or, to give it the proper term, coagulation. It would be impossible to deal with all the clotting factors in a book of this length, so I shall instead describe a few of the key components and explain how they fit the coagulation jigsaw.

THE PLATELETS

These disc-shaped structures are found in the blood of all mammals. As well as their beneficial function in preventing us bleeding to death when we are injured, platelets also play a major role in atherosclerosis and thrombosis. Platelets are formed in the bone marrow, and there is normally a consistent number of them circulating in the bloodstream.

The outer membrane of the platelet is of critical importance to the control of a process called haemostasis. When functioning normally, haemostasis prevents blood loss from intact, undamaged vessels and stops excessive bleeding from cut blood vessels. In other words, haemostasis is a control system which allows blood to clot only when necessary.

The platelet membrane is thought to be the source of a substance called platelet factor 3 which, when released by the platelet, accelerates blood clotting. Under normal conditions, the circulating platelets do not mass together to form clumps, nor do they stick to the lining of the blood vessels. However, when these linings are damaged, the circulating platelets become sticky, aggregating at the site of the injury and, together with the other blood coagulation factors, forming a clot or plug to arrest the bleeding. This process is haemostasis.

At this point, it is worth mentioning certain substances secreted by the arteries during the platelet activation process. A normal artery releases thromboxane A2 when damage occurs; this stimulates the platelets to clump together to stop the bleeding. But, to prevent any unnecessary, excessive clotting, the artery also releases prostacyclin. Unfortunately, in damaged arteries which have developed atheroma, it appears that prostacyclin is not released, thus compounding the problem of atheroma.

As the process of atheroma progresses, a layer of cells spreads over it. This does not happen by chance, but is instigated by another product of the platelet – the growth factor. This factor encourages the lining cells of the vessel wall to proliferate and grow over the atheroma. When this process has been repeated numerous times, the result is a blocked artery.

The Use of Garlic to Counteract Platelet Stickiness

Eating garlic and onions can reverse undesirable platelet stickiness. Let's take a look at some of the studies which demonstrate this useful effect.

Back in 1972, Dr Weisenberger and colleagues reported that onion, when tested in the laboratory, inhibited platelet aggregation. This was very interesting, but proof of its efficacy had to be demonstrated in humans before any anti-clotting virtues could be claimed. What was most useful about this study was the identification of the inhibitor as a substance called adenosine. However, other researchers pointed out that adenosine could not possibly be the responsible compound because it was not absorbed from the gastrointestinal tract. Later, it was suggested that garlic contains unknown compounds which allow adenosine to pass through the cell barriers which line the gastrointestinal tract.

When one eats a meal containing a high proportion of fat, there is a tendency for the platelets to aggregate more readily. Dr Baghurst and colleagues tested this on a number of patients and published their results in the *Lancet* in 1977. These researchers fed patients a meal with a high saturated fat content similar to the one I describe in my triglyceride study, and they also added 75 grams of fried onion to the meal. It was discovered that the platelets stuck together far less readily.

In another study, Professor Bordia demonstrated that, in blood drawn from healthy adults, the platelets could be made to aggregate by chemical means. But, if oil of garlic was given to the patients before the blood samples were taken, aggregation did not occur.

Thrombosis in Horses

A patient who regularly visited farms in France told me this story. It seems that horses, too, have circulation problems – they are susceptible to thrombosis of the leg arteries, which gives them considerable pain and can lead to death. However, French farmers have a remedy: if the horses are fed quantities of garlic and onion, the clots gradually disappear and leave the animals fit and active.

FIBRINOGEN

The clot formed by the platelets sticking together is at first quite fragile, and must be reinforced. This is where the vitally important protein called fibrinogen comes in. Again, it is a matter of having the correct concentration of fibrinogen in the blood – too much can lead to acceleration of clot formation. As we get older, many people acquire a higher level of fibrinogen. This seems to apply particularly to those who are prone to heart attacks. Smokers, also, have a tendency to high fibrinogen levels – another excellent reason for kicking the habit.

BLOOD VISCOSITY

If the viscosity of the blood is increased – in other words, if the flow becomes thicker, and therefore slower – there is an increased tendency to heart attacks. It is possible to reduce the blood viscosity by eating more oily fish and reducing the intake of saturated fat. Garlic has a similar effect.

Onions to the Rescue

In the late 1960s, when I was just starting my research and was faced with scepticism and negative reactions, an article appeared in a medical journal which described the effect of onions on the blood circulation of a group of hospital patients suffering from coronary artery disease. The patients were being treated with anticoagulant drugs to 'thin' their blood and stop undesirable clotting. What the researchers found was that replacing the drug with onion had precisely the same effect. I had a conversation with one of the research team, who said that it had been possible to withdraw the anticoagulant drug because the onion was doing the work as efficiently, and in a natural manner. Just think how much more effective the treatment would have been if the patients had taken garlic.

At this point, I must warn against anyone stopping their blood 'thinning' treatment in favour of garlic. Listen to your doctor – he or she knows the best treatment for you. By all means, take a garlic oil capsule daily and have garlic in your diet – the former will do nothing but good, and the latter will give you more enjoyment from your food. But regard garlic as a healthy extra rather than a substitute, unless you receive professional medical advice to stop taking your drug.

Triglycerides are Linked with Clotting

This was the opportunity I had been waiting for. Here was convincing evidence that garlic and onion could be of great benefit to mankind, with a distinct possibility of saving a huge number of lives. One of my medical colleagues became interested in my theories and, at last, I was able to put my ideas into practice.

In 1968, very few people in the UK – particularly in Sheffield – would have dreamed of eating garlic. It was regarded as some sort of foreign muck with a disgusting smell and even worse after-effects. Certainly, our patients were unlikely to agree to eat several cloves of garlic with their traditional high-fat breakfast, and garlic capsules were not readily available. But I still needed to test my theory, so I decided to ask the patients whether they would find onion acceptable.

Much to my delight, sixteen men, all of whom had suffered a heart attack, volunteered for the study. The patients agreed to have two breakfasts: one with raw, boiled or fried onion, and the other without, several days apart. The breakfast, consisting of bacon, fried egg, cornflakes and cream, toast and butter, and milk to drink, contained a lot of fat. After the meal, on each occasion I tested the patients' blood triglyceride levels. To my joy, I found that, when onion was also included in the breakfast, it partially prevented the rise in triglycerides which occurs after such a high-fat meal.

RED BLOOD CELLS

The red blood cells which circulate through all our arteries and veins carry the vital oxygen to our organs. The successful transfer of oxygen to the tissues and carbon dioxide from them relies on the outer membrane or envelope of the cell being flexible and deformable. This allows the red cells to pass along capillary blood vessels which are much smaller in diameter than they are.

Clearly, if the cells are more rigid they will not only be unable to pass down the capillaries to complete the exchange of gases, but will actually block the vessel, causing serious problems.

Some people with heart disease have these more rigid red blood cells, particularly if their diet is rich in saturated animal fats. Until I researched the material for this book I thought the oils from fish, which I researched for many years, were the only way to help make the red cells more flexible. Now, I strongly suspect that garlic has the same effect.

Improved Circulation with Garlic

There is now evidence that, over a four-week period on garlic powder, the viscosity of the blood can actually decrease by 3.2 per cent – a small but important change in the right direction. As a result of this change, and an inhibition of platelet aggregation, the red blood cells are able to pass freely through the microcirculation – the body's network of extremely fine-bore arteries and veins. An improvement in the microcirculation in turn

---

A Personal Experience

Many stories have reached my ears about the effectiveness of garlic in improving the circulation. Numerous people, most of them elderly, have told me this tale and I must say that I have been rather sceptical. However, when I took my first garlic oil capsule immediately before breakfast I experienced a warming sensation which, I must admit, was quite pleasant. Obviously, it was impossible for me to state categorically that this effect was due to garlic, although for the life of me I could not believe that my toast and marmalade were responsible. Like any good researcher, I decided to take the capsules at different times of day, with food and without food. Lo and behold, they achieved the same effect.

improved the circulation to the hands, feet and surface of the body. These changes were first reported by Dr H. Kiesewetter and his colleagues in 1991 in the *International Journal of Clinical Pharmacology, Therapy and Toxicology*.

FIBRINOLYTIC ACTIVITY

After the platelets have formed a plug to stem the flow of blood, the clot is consolidated by fibrin, the final product in the process. Although this stabilises the platelet plug in just a few minutes, the fibrin carries on its work and eventually forms a fibrin plug.

To allow the vessel wall to heal effectively, the fibrin must be removed to allow the cells which normally cover the vessel wall to cover the wound. This process, known as fibrinolytic activity, dissolves the clot effectively. However, in many older people and those with abnormally high blood fat levels, the fibrinolytic activity is reduced. This is particularly noticeable in patients with high blood triglyceride. In these people, the clots do not dissolve, but build up and become part of the clogging process in the arteries. Ultimately, this leads to angina or a heart attack.

Garlic, Onion and Fibrinolytic Activity

In 1966, Dr Gupta performed a study on patients similar to the one which I undertook a year or two later. He took blood samples from patients in the fasting state, and then at intervals after a fatty breakfast containing 60 grams of fried onion. One would expect the fibrinolytic activity to decrease after a fatty meal – in other words, the tendency to dissolve clots would be impaired. But what Dr Gupta found was an increase.

The findings of several similar projects were reported relatively soon after Dr Gupta's research. They all examined the effects of dried, boiled, fried and raw onions on fibrinolytic activity and, in each case, an increase was experienced.

Subsequent to these onion studies, it was found that garlic oil or garlic juice had similar benefits.

Here's some good news for older people, whose fibrinolytic activity is likely to be decreasing. Dr Jain had found that feeding 100 grams of onion to patients before testing their fibrinolytic acctivity had greater beneficial effects on older people than on the young.

There is just one further piece of research which is worth mentioning here – a study by Professor Bordia which was reported in the international journal *Atherosclerosis* in 1977. Essential oil of garlic was administered to forty volunteers who included ten healthy subjects, ten patients with a history of old myocardial infarction (heart attacks) and twenty patients with acute myocardial infarction. Over a three-month period, their fibrinolytic activity was consistently raised, only falling when the treatment was stopped.

What was most interesting was that the patients with acute myocardial infarction also experienced increased fibrinolytic activity. The important point here was that these patients were in hospital recovering from a heart attack. It is well known that if fibrinolytic activity cannot be increased during the crucial period just after an attack, the patient is likely to suffer another attack due to the development of further blood clots.

GARLIC, ASPIRIN AND FISH OIL

Low-dose aspirin has been prescribed for a number of years as an anti-platelet drug in the treatment of heart disease and strokes. Its effect is to increase what is known as the bleeding time, by reducing the stickiness of the platelets. In this way, excessive clot formation can be controlled.

In order to measure a patient's bleeding time, two incisions are made in the forearm, each 5mm long by 1mm deep and avoiding any large blood vessels. The incisions are blotted every thirty seconds with filter paper until the bleeding stops. The bleeding time is the time it takes for bleeding to stop – usually between two and ten minutes.

A Lick Is All it Takes

This test has its faults but, apart from criticisms of its accuracy which pop up at regular intervals, is a generally accepted method of measuring bleeding. The dose of aspirin generally used to increase the bleeding time is 75mg daily. In 1981, I attended a conference in Toronto at which the late Professor J.R.A. Mitchell stated that the daily dose required to prevent platelets sticking together was no more than a single lick of an aspirin tablet.

Does Aspirin Cause Problems?

About 1 per cent of patients taking aspirin to control clotting suffer from significant internal bleeding caused by the irritant effect of the drug. For their sake, we need to look for a replacement for aspirin. It may be that, after further research, fish oil or garlic, both of which seem to have few, if any, adverse side-effects, may prove to be the answer.

Fish Oil and Bleeding Time

In 1990 I chaired a meeting of a group of international experts convened to discuss the effects of fish and fish oil on the bleeding time, and any interaction between this and aspirin. Obviously, if both aspirin and fish oil prolonged bleeding time, there was a real possibility that, if both were taken together, excessive bleeding might result.

I looked at almost one hundred scientific papers reporting studies on the effect of fish and fish oil on the bleeding time. With one or two exceptions, the bleeding time was increased, suggesting a beneficial effect on platelets, and thus reducing the risk of clot formation.

The opinion of the group was that aspirin could be given at

the same time as fish oil without any harmful effects, provided that not too much fish oil was taken. An intake of 2 to 3 grams daily of the omega 3 fatty acids present in fish did not cause any problems when taken with aspirin.

Does Garlic Have a Similar Effect?

As far as I am aware, no major study to compare the efficacy of garlic with that of aspirin in the field of clot prevention has yet been undertaken. Readers of this book will have been aware by now that many studies have shown that, in both humans and animals, the sulphur compounds in garlic act as effective inhibitors of platelet stickiness. There is absolutely no reason why garlic should not prove to be just as effective as aspirin in this role, and much safer. Indeed, I would recommend everyone to take garlic, fresh or in capsules, together with their daily dose of fish oil, to help keep a healthy heart and circulation.

Future Research

What is needed now is a large-scale study to compare the effects of garlic, fish oil and aspirin in the prevent of first and subsequent heart attacks. This study should take in as large a number of patients as possible, and should continue for several years. As I have already point out, coronary disease develops over many years, usually revealing itself in the patient's forties, fifties or sixties. In a disease with such a long incubation period, studies of a few weeks are nothing more than an indicator of what might happen with a particular treatment. Only time will tell.

High Blood Pressure

Many people suffer from high blood pressure, and it is one of the most important risk factors for heart attack. The conventional treatment with drugs must account for a large slice of the NHS budget. Yet a large number of studies have shown that blood pressure can be reduced by including more garlic in our diet, or by taking a garlic oil supplement.

In a normal adult, the upper limit of acceptable blood pressure varies with age. Any pressure of 160/95 or higher is considered abnormal and referred to as hypertension. The higher of the two figures is known as the systolic blood pressure, and the lower as the diastolic blood pressure. Nowadays, the diastolic pressure is regarded as the more useful indication of blood pressure because, in older people, the systolic cannot be significantly reduced. The reason for this is that, with age, the walls of the arteries, and especially the aorta leading from the heart, become hardened and lose their elasticity. They are therefore less able to stretch and absorb some of the pressure changes caused when the heart pumps blood through the circulation, and high blood pressure can result.

LABILE HYPERTENSION

In people who suffer stress due to their work or lifestyle, a condition known as Gaisbock's syndrome, or labile hypertension, can occur. This simply means that the blood pressure varies from high to low, which can be a precursor of permanent hypertension. If the person's lifestyle does become more relaxed, the blood pressure remains high and becomes an important risk factor for the development of a heart attack.

One of the problems with hypertension is that the sufferer is often unaware of it until he or she visits the doctor for a routine examination. It is then important to receive treatment, which often consists of drugs. Among the commonest are the beta blockers, which reduce the blood pressure and heart rate, but also slow the person down. Tiredness is a common side-effect of the beta blockers. These drugs are not recommended in patients suffering from respiratory problems such as asthma; for them another type of drug, the calcium channel blocker, is used.

Earlier in this chapter I described how the heart pumped blood through the body by contracting and relaxing. In order to do this, it requires a number of chemicals, one of which is calcium. However, when someone has angina or hypertension, or has suffered a heart attack, it is usual to try to reduce the work of the heart muscle in an attempt to protect it and prevent it overworking. This is where the calcium channel blockers come in, by partially blocking the movement of calcium into the cells of the heart muscle. A slowing down of the heart rate follows, and there is a bonus, dilating effect on the arteries.

All drugs, however, have side-effects, and are expensive.

SALT AND HYPERTENSION

We tend to eat food which has been liberally laced with table salt because it improves the flavour and we have become used to the taste. We actually need about one gram of salt a day for our bodies to function normally. On average, we consume ten times this amount. The majority of us can cope with this much salt, but the remainder – people with liver disease, kidney problems and certain forms of heart disease – cannot. The result is high blood pressure.

The amount of salt that we sprinkle on our food is really quite small – most of those 10 grams come from ready-prepared foods, or are added to our food during cooking. A bag of ready-salted potato crisps is a good example, and many packet foods, such as soups, contain more salt than necessary. I find that if my meals contain garlic the food has sufficient flavour for me not to need the salt.

LOWERING BLOOD PRESSURE

It is a good idea to have our blood pressure checked periodically as we get older. Once a year is sufficient. Some people believe they have high blood pressure because they suffer headaches and have dizzy spells. But this does not usually happen in mild hypertension, and the headaches are probably due to some other cause.

Look, first of all, at your family history. A history of hypertension among your relatives should send you to your doctor for a blood pressure check. You can help yourself by reducing the amount of salt you eat. Also, if you have a stressful life, you should look at ways of relaxing more and exercising. You may even find some sort of meditation helpful, either alone or with a group. If you do have raised blood pressure, your doctor will probably prescribe some form of medication. It will do no harm, and will probably help, if you also take fresh garlic or garlic capsules every day. But note that world 'also': you must take whatever medication is prescribed as well.

The Great Smokies Trail

Many scientific studies have been carried out on the effect of garlic on blood pressure. In order to persuade you of its benefits, I can do no better than bring to your attention a paper published in 1987 by Dr S.A. Barrie and colleagues from the Great Smokies Medical Center in North Carolina. In the preceding research study, the authors tested garlic oil on twenty healthy human volunteers. All the volunteers were students, and their average age was twenty-six. Before participating in the study, the volunteers were asked to avoid any drugs which interfered with platelet aggregation, and to limit the amount of garlic in their meals.

Over a four-week period during which their diet was supplemented with garlic oil, their average blood pressure fell significantly when compared with a similar-length placebo period. The placebo in this case was a dummy capsule containing a substance which could have no effect on blood pressure. You might say that the volunteers would know which capsule contained the garlic because of its smell, and that this might have some effect – but not in this particular study. The researchers were careful to ensure that the placebo capsule, too, had that distinctive garlic odour!

3

ON THE BRINK OF NEW DISCOVERIES

A Natural Antibiotic

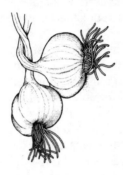

Before launching into a description of how the onion family, and garlic in particular, can be harnessed to fight infection, I want to say a few words about the living organisms responsible for causing some of the diseases to which humans can fall victim. These organisms can be called bacteria, micro-organisms or just plain 'bugs'.

PATHOGENS AND NON-PATHOGENS

Bacteria come in two varieties. Pathogens, which are capable of producing disease in the human host, and non-pathogens, which are not. Many non-pathogenic bacteria live in and on us, playing vital roles in keeping our bodies functioning properly. For instance, there are bacteria living in our gastrointestinal tract which help to break down and digest our food. Without these bacteria, we would probably die from malnutrition.

The non-pathogenic bacteria resident in our bodies also help to keep some of the pathogenic bacteria at bay, by destroying enough to maintain the correct balance. (However, things can go wrong and, in some circumstances, even the non-pathogens can cause infection.)

When you are taking antibiotics, have you ever noticed the change in size and consistency of your faeces? This is usually due to the destruction of the non-pathogens, and can be an unwanted and uncomfortable side-effect. In the early 1960s, it was found that taking the antibiotic neomycin resulted in a dramatic fall in the blood fats. After much discussion and argument, it was concluded that this was due to the removal of the resident bacteria. This resulted in the body's failure to absorb essential food products. This was all right in the short term and, who knows, may have helped people to lose some weight. But it was asking for trouble to use it for any length of time. I believe there are now stringent restrictions on the use of neomycin.

Another point about bacteria is their ability to adapt to changing conditions. Conventional antibiotics are extremely useful drugs in the treatment of many infections, ranging from a simple sore throat to serious, life-threatening conditions. But one drawback to their use is the ability of the infecting organism to become resistant to the antibiotic.

Garlic Versus Bacteria

Moving on to the garlic effect, you may remember I talked earlier about Albert Schweitzer using garlic to treat chronic dysentery. Also how, during the First World War, the Russian Army used it as a cure for gangrene. In the absence of conventional antibiotics, garlic seemed to be very effective, and free from the problems associated with antibiotics.

In 1856, one of the world's greatest scientists, Louis Pasteur, wrote at length about garlic in a French scientific journal. Pasteur was internationally famous for his spectacular discoveries of the organisms – and the vaccines against them – that caused the killer diseases anthrax and rabies. If Pasteur was convinced of the power of garlic, I think we must take the matter very seriously indeed.

A century later, in 1956 and 1957, scientific papers were published on the efficiency of certain herbs and spices in destroying several of the organisms responsible for food poisoning. Garlic was the only herb which effectively dealt with the organisms *Shigella sonnei*, *Staphylococcus aureus*, *Escherichia coli*, *Streptococcus faecalis* and *Lactobacillus casei*, all of which are capable of causing serious health problems.

In 1985, Dr G.R. Fenwick and Dr A.B. Hanley published an excellent paper in the CRC Critical Reviews in *Food Science and Nutrition*, volume 22, entitled 'The Genus Allium', which ably described the antibacterial effects of garlic and onions. The authors list twenty-three species of organisms which have been reported by various scientists to be inhibited by the alliums. In 1993 a two year study was commenced. Due to be published in 1995 it was carried out at the University of Wolverhampton by Ms Zara Ross as part of her Ph.D. thesis. Supervised by Dr. David Hill, Senior Lecturer in Microbiology, the study used human gut fluids to look at the effects of steam distilled essential oils of garlic (Cardiomax) on several important and problematic bacteria. The key organisms (Salmonella

enteritides and Listeria monocytogenes) have both been implicated in recent times in outbreaks of food poisoning arising from
eggs, chickens and unpasturised soft cheeses. Listeria m. was
found to be remarkably sensitive to Garlic oil and easily controlled by it and Salmonella also required only minute traces of
the oil in gut fluid to be eradicated. A very important further
finding was that commensal bacteria which inhabit the human
intestine and are valuable to gastro-intestinal health, were not
unduly affected by the bactericidal effects of garlic oil whereas
anti-biotic controls might well have exerted an adverse effect.

FUNGAL AND YEAST INFECTIONS OF THE BODY

There are many irritating and persistent fungal and yeast infections which affect humans, including athlete's foot, cystitis,
thrush, ringworm and vaginitis.

Thrush, if untreated, can lead to a number of serious conditions, and may even affect blood glucose levels. But it can be
difficult to treat, often because the organism has become resistant to antibiotics used previously. Personal cleanliness and high
doses of garlic (several cloves or capsules of garlic oil taken by
mouth) can help to treat this condition.

Ringworm is still around today. It is fairly common in pets
and may be passed on, for example, by a dog trimmer who is not
scrupulous about sterilising instruments. Garlic is an ideal treatment, and can be used on the skin as well as being taken by
mouth.

Cancer Prevention

Responsible for one in four deaths in the UK, cancer is, understandably, an emotive subject. So, before anyone accuses me of
making too many claims, I must reiterate that garlic is not

a cure-all or miracle herb. Secondly, the garlic and cancer research that I am aware of at the time of writing is based on both animal and human work, with the emphasis on animals. These initial findings need close examination, and the research must be extended to concentrate more on humans before we can say for certain whether garlic has a role to play in the fight against cancer.

WHAT IS CANCER?

When most people speak of cancer, they seem to refer to a single disease. However, there are, in fact, many different forms of it. Common types include cancer of the bladder, prostate gland, breast, lung, skin, colon, rectum and stomach. Leukaemia is also regarded as a form of cancer.

There are different levels and stages in cancer development, and conventional treatment by radiotherapy, chemotherapy or surgery can be given either individually or collectively – with success in many patients.

Our body cells increase in number when we are young and still growing, until the in-built control mechanisms decide that enough is enough. But, even when we have finished growing, many organs, notably the skin, continue to renew old cells throughout our lives. Quite normal tissues need to discard old cells and replace them with new ones – this is part of maintaining a healthy, efficient body. As an example, the bone marrow, which is responsible for producing blood, needs to replace 2,000 million red blood cells every day.

How Cancer Strikes

If a group of cells is no longer under the control of the system responsible for their proper renewal, a tumour starts to develop. As the tumour, or cancer, grows it can invade and destroy surrounding tissues. Groups of cancer cells can break off into the bloodstream, where they are carried round the body to start their work elsewhere.

GARLIC: THE EVIDENCE SO FAR

Many chemicals in daily use have the ability to trigger cancer growth. Skin, liver and lung cancer are but three which can be instigated by chemicals somewhere in our environment. It may be that these substances are used in our work, or appear in our food supply.

In New York, a group of researchers, Dr Belman, Dr Block and Dr Barany, produced skin cancers in mice by using some of these chemicals. They decided to see if garlic oil could prevent the further development of cancers, and found that it did. Although this research has only been carried out on animals, it is a promising beginning and it is to be hoped that further research and results will follow.

Garlic: A Review of its Relationship to Cancer, is the title of a publication by Dr Sumiyoshi and Dr Wargovitch. These researchers reviewed the current evidence of garlic's ability to prevent certain chemicals inducing cancer. They used the same carcinogenic chemicals as those of the New York study. (A carcinogen is a substance which, when in contact with human or animal bodies, can trigger the cancer process). These authors summed up their review in the following terms: 'The precise inhibitory mechanism of garlic on carcinogenesis has not yet been characterised, [but] constituents of garlic are slowly being revealed to be excellent experimental inhibitors of both the initiating and promoting phases of carcinogenesis.'

In plain language, this means that some substances in garlic prevent cancer starting its terrible work, and may even arrest established cancers. This is a bold assessment, in my opinion, but it has been made on the authors' interpretation of published research, which they have carefully considered.

In 1989, Dr Jang and his co-workers were able to instigate pre-cancerous changes in rat livers by giving the animals the chemical diethylnitrosamine, a known carcinogen. Again, garlic demonstrated beneficial effects at this early stage. A Japanese research group came up with similar results in mice.

In *Cancer Research*, 1988, Dr M.J. Wargovitch and colleagues from the University of Texas reported the results of using a chemical carcinogen to produce cancer of the oesophagus in rats. The oesophagus is the large tube through which all our food passes. It starts at the back of the mouth, and stops at the entry to the stomach. Cancer of the oesophagus is not uncommon in humans, but it is difficult to treat.

The rats that were given the carcinogen developed cancerous lesions of the oesophagus. Those rats that were given the carcinogen *and* diallyl sulphide, a by-product of garlic, developed no such lesions. The implications are exciting, but only when humans replace rats will we know if garlic really can have such a dramatic effect.

Research involving garlic and gastric cancer was carried out by Dr W.C. You and colleagues at the Beijing Institute for Cancer Research in the People's Republic of China. The results were published in 1989 in the *Journal of the National Cancer Institute* under the title 'Allium Vegetables and Reduced Risk of Stomach Cancer'. This study was particularly interesting because it was based on humans rather than animals, and was carried out in a part of China in which gastric cancer was prevalent.

Two groups of people were interviewed, the first comprising 564 with stomach cancer, and the second 1,131 with no evidence of the disease. The research revealed a significant reduction in the incidence of stomach cancer in relation to increased consumption of *Allium* vegetables. The subjects who had the highest *Allium* consumption, mainly onion and garlic, ran only 40 per cent of the risk of developing gastric cancer, compared to those who ate the least. This impressive paper will, it is hoped, be followed up by further research on humans.

Moving on five years, in 1994 a study was reported in *Carcinogenesis* by Dr X.Y. Lin, Dr J.Z. Lui and Dr J.A. Milner in which n-nitroso compounds (NOCs) were given to rats. Members of this group of substances have been implicated in the development of numerous animal cancers. Although there is no absolutely firm evidence that NOCs are responsible for cancer in humans, it is important to establish their role because they are present in the environment and in our food and drink. It is possible that they cause damage to the DNA in our genes, with serious consequences.

The synthesis of NOCs in the body can be partially inhibited by vitamin C, and the trial was designed to establish a similar role for garlic powder when fed to affected rats. When 2 per cent garlic was added to the rats' diet, the presence of the carcinogenic substances in their tissue was reduced by over 50 per cent. When the garlic dose was increased to 4 per cent, the reduction was around 70 per cent.

Radiation and Garlic

We hear a lot about radiation, in connection not only with nuclear bombs, but also with the use of nuclear power to provide cheap electricity. In fact, natural radiation is all around us. It can be found in the landscape. In some areas of Britain, for example, rocks give off radon, a radioactive gas. The sun also bombards us with radiation. This does not cause widespread problems in countries with little strong sun, even though there is now a hole in the ozone layer. In hot countries, however, or if we expose ourselves too much to the sun's rays, skin cancer can develop. If this happens to humans, think what would happen to microscopic organisms; they would quickly die.

Dr Knasmulle and his colleagues in Innsbruck, Austria, subjected two types of micro-organisms to lethal doses of gamma irradiation. The researchers were excited to find that a property in garlic was able to reduce the potentially lethal effects of this radiation. The organisms used in the study were *Escherichia coli* and *Salmonella typhimurium*, both of which we would normally be delighted to destroy. However, they proved to be good experimental material and indicated that, as ever, we should conduct more garlic research on humans.

Garlic Against Free Radicals

WHAT ARE FREE RADICALS?

Substances called antioxidants are much in the news these days, and in this section I shall explain why they are necessary for health. But to start with, I ought to say what free radicals are, since the two have a close relationship.

During our normal activities, the food we consume and the oxygen we breathe are constantly utilised by the body as fuel for its cells. When the food is converted into energy or used to repair the body cells, carbon dioxide, water and waste are the by-products. It is from these waste products that the oxidising agents, which we know as free radicals, are produced. Obviously, the processes which produce them are going on every moment of day and night. Therefore, free radicals are constantly being released.

Cell Damage

The free radicals are unstable materials, and can attack the molecules of the body cells. They contribute to many of the degenerative diseases which affect humans, and are considered to be an important factor in the process of accelerated ageing.

How Do Free Radicals Affect the Heart?

Free radicals can have a damaging effect on the coronary arteries. When I discussed cholesterol in Chapter 2, I pointed out that a certain amount was necessary for a healthy body, but that an excess of low-density lipoprotein, or LDL, was harmful.

When the cells of the arteries take up cholesterol normally, the amount utilised is rigidly controlled. However, if excessive levels of free radical are available, the LDL cholesterol oxidises and damages the artery walls. It may be just as important to protect LDL against the attentions of free radicals as it is to reduce cholesterol levels in the blood.

Other Conditions Arising from Free Radical Attack

A number of other pathological conditions, some of them very major indeed, are associated with free radical attack. They include auto-immune disease, cancer, drug toxicity (a kind of side-effect of drugs), surgical trauma, and diabetes (see page 73-74).

ANTIOXIDANTS

Now into the arena rides the arch-enemy of free radicals, the antioxidants. In our diet we take in a certain amount of antioxidants in the form of vitamin E, vitamin C and beta-carotene, which are sometimes described as the antioxidant vitamins. The foods which contain the antioxidants include fresh fruit and vegetables, but vitamin E comes mainly in nuts.

A Warning About Nuts

Although nuts are a good source of vitamin E, I have strong reservations about recommending them. Unfortunately, some people have a very strong allergy to nuts. There has been considerable publicity regarding the dangers of peanut allergy, which can sometimes be fatal. Less well known is an allergy to walnuts, which can make the sufferer's mouth swell so much that he or she finds it difficult to breathe. If you have this type of allergy, do as I do and take your vitamin E in capsule form.

Vitamin E deficiency is not a problem in human beings. In fact, although the US government states a minimum daily allowance, the British government does not. Any food containing polyunsaturated fats appears to contain vitamin E to protect its fats against oxidation. I feel my daily vitamin E capsule, together with vitamin C and selenium, help to protect my body against free radical attack. This may seem a belt-and-braces approach, but it is certainly not doing me any harm.

WHERE DOES GARLIC FIT IN?

Garlic is thought to neutralise the free radicals, and there is some evidence of its ability to destroy oxidising agents in body cells. The body cells are complicated structures containing components known as microsomes, which have a fat-based membrane and can only be seen using ultra-microscopic techniques.

In 1989, a paper was published in *Planta Medica* by a group of Japanese researchers led by Dr T. Horie. He and his colleagues had conducted experiments in which the livers of rats were exposed to free radicals. As I have stated throughout this book, when discussing the results of scientific research it is difficult to transfer results on animals to man. Nevertheless, it was most heartening to read that, in this study, garlic proved effective in preventing some of the chemical and physical changes which one would have expected to find.

In a review on garlic in the prevention and treatment of cardiovascular disease published in the journal *Phytotherapy* in 1993, Dr H.D. Reuter talks about the initial process in the development of atherosclerosis – the formation of foam cells in the artery walls by the uptake of oxidised LDL cholesterol. This author reports a number of human and animal studies in which the deposition of LDL cholesterol in the vessel wall may be prevented by garlic.

It seems to me that garlic is a relatively cheap, readily available and seemingly effective weapon against the assault on our bodies by free radicals and other undesirable substances.

To consume garlic regularly, or take it as a dietary supplement, can do nothing but good. I shall continue to eat fresh garlic and to take my Cardiomax garlic oil capsule each day – and I would recommend readers to do the same.

Diabetes

The ancient literature on the medicinal properties of garlic describes its use in the treatment of diabetes – a condition characterised by excessive blood glucose. I do not recommend garlic at the present time (although it can do no harm), but in the course of time, and after more research, a place may be found for it alongside present conventional methods of reducing blood glucose.

GARLIC VERSUS CONVENTIONAL THERAPY

The principal drug used throughout the world to treat diabetes is called tolbutamide. It works by lowering the blood sugar. When researchers gave garlic and onion extracts to animals, the blood sugar-reducing effect was shown to be close to that of tolbutamide. Some researchers suggest that garlic contains a component which prevents a rise in blood sugar after the consumption of sugar-rich foods.

INSULIN PRODUCTION

Earlier, I described how the triglycerides in the blood are raised after a meal. There is a similar effect on the blood glucose level in these circumstances. The blood glucose is controlled by insulin, a hormone produced by the pancreas. Insulin is released in response to increased levels of glucose in the blood. Diabetics are unable to produce sufficient insulin to deal with the blood glucose rise; without treatment, the consequences are severe.

The degree of the rise in blood glucose, measured over a period of several hours, indicates the efficiency of an individual's insulin release. A group of researchers tested the effect of four different doses of onion extract on healthy human volunteers. They found that the blood glucose reduced in proportion to the size of the onion dose, and occurred after the volunteers had been given the extract together with glucose. Their blood glucose was unaffected when they had not eaten a meal with the onion extract.

4

GARLIC REMEDIES FOR EVERYDAY AILMENTS

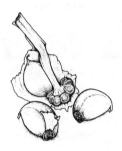

Talk about any subject concerned with human health, and there are always dozens of old wives' tales to go with it. Garlic is no exception; in this case, however, the tales are often based on fact. This chapter gives a selection of useful garlic remedies which, although not proved by carefully designed experiments, have nevertheless been found effective. (See also page 64, which lists some fungal infections that can be alleviated with garlic.)

Colds and Flu

These are the result of virus infections which cannot be cured through treatment with antibiotics. The only thing we can hope to do is to alleviate some of the unpleasant symptoms, such as sneezing and generally feeling rotten.

One way of doing this is to take garlic in milk. Place several cloves of garlic, sliced or crushed, in about a third of a pint (200ml) of milk, bring to the boil and simmer for a few minutes. Drink while still warm.

The unpleasant congestion that often accompanies a cold can be relieved by heating a lot of garlic or onion in a little water and inhaling the vapour.

Sinusitis

The decongestant remedy given above works well for blocked sinuses – garlic contains a particular chemical which makes mucus runny.

Sore Throats and Coughs

If you need something to soothe a sore throat, try this remedy. It is equally effective for the persistent cough that sometimes remains when other cold or flu symptoms have disappeared.

Slice three or four garlic cloves and place them in a covered container together with three tablespoons of honey. Leave for three to four hours, and take as required on a spoon.

Earache

I once read of an earache remedy which, although effective, left doubts in my mind about its safety. It consisted of simply placing a warmed garlic clove in the offending ear.

I would never recommend this method, but would suggest the

following instead. Heat a sliced garlic clove in a little olive oil. Strain the cooled oil, and pour it into the ear. The oil is more effective if it is still warm (but not hot!). Alternatively, warm the oil from a garlic oil capsule and use it in the same way.

NB: persistent earache can have a variety of causes and requires examination by a doctor.

Spots and Boils

To destroy spots, rub them with a small slice of garlic. If the spot is infected, or if you have a boil, a strong concoction of crushed garlic in honey, applied at regular intervals, will give relief.

It is interesting that honey is often used as the 'carrier' for garlic remedies. For many years, a mixture of honey and cod-liver oil was used in hospital for treating leg ulcers.

Acne

This distressing condition frequently affects the skin of teenagers. At the base of the hair follicles, from which hair grows, are sebaceous glands which produce an oily substance called sebum. Hormonal upheaval during adolescence can cause overproduction of sebum, resulting in the glands becoming blocked. Groups of spots or pimples then appear on the back and face.

A good diet with plenty of fresh fruit and vegetables can be helpful, but the usual treatment recommended is a long course of antibiotics. Before embarking on this course of action, which is expensive and probably not without certain side-effects, it is worth trying the garlic treatment. As well as taking liberal quantities of garlic in your diet, there are two ways of treating the spots themselves.

The first method involves a face mask consisting of a mixture of garlic, honey and kaolin power. Blend three chopped cloves of garlic with a dessertspoonful (10ml) of runny honey and a tablespoon of kaolin power (obtainable from the chemist). Apply to the affected area, keeping the mixture away from your eyes.

The other method is to blend three or four chopped garlic cloves with about 8fl.oz (225ml) of surgical spirit. Keep the mixture in a stoppered glass container in the refrigerator and dab it daily on to the affected areas. As before, keep the mixture away from your eyes.

Warts and Veruccas

When I was at school, veruccas were a fairly common infection of the feet, usually contracted in the showers. At that time, treatment consisted of regular X-rays of the affected areas – this was long before the potential dangers of multiple X-rays was appreciated.

To treat either veruccas or warts, first protect the surrounding skin with vaseline. Then cut a small slice of fresh garlic and apply it to the offending excrescence. Cover with a plaster, and change daily until the verucca or wart can be lifted out.

Athlete's Foot

This condition is caused by a fungal infection and results in soreness, irritation, and embarrassment! Treat it with olive oil in which you have immersed some crushed garlic for a day or two. Use this garlic oil two or three times a day until the problem clears.

Garlic as a Mosquito Repellent

You may remember my earlier story of the children who had trouble with mosquitoes in Italy. The child who took a garlic capsule every day was untouched, but his more obstinate brother, who took no garlic, was bitten all over. The moral is obvious!

Parasites and Intestinal Worms

How I wish I had known about garlic several years ago when I did a lecture tour of India. Despite taking care, I contracted a severe intestinal infection which had to be treated with a drug called metronidazole. In some ways, the effect of the drug was as bad as the original infection! We now know, however, that garlic is effective against amoebic dysentery.

While amoebic dysentery can hardly be called an everyday ailment in Britain, garlic has always been the enemy of all manner of intestinal worms. The sulphides which it produces attack the parasites and allow them to be expelled from the body. Research has shown that, when garlic is taken, types of worms that reside in the higher levels of the gastrointestinal tract are killed and expelled.

Sprains

Crush two or three cloves of garlic and mix thoroughly with a little olive oil. When this mixture is applied to the sprain and covered with a dressing, it is reputed to give some pain relief and to reduce the swelling.

Arthritis

Some relief from the pain of arthritis can be obtained by massaging the affected area with a mixture of one part crushed garlic to nine parts of olive oil.

Indigestion and Diarrhoea

Using garlic in your diet seems to give some protection against indigestion – I certainly find it helps. I have already mentioned the value of garlic in dealing effectively with food poisoning. This remedy is also effective against diarrhoea, but if the condition persists you must consult your doctor.

Piles and Varicose Veins

Both these conditions are similar, consisting of veins which have become engorged with blood and hardened with thrombosed areas. In Chapter 2 I explained the usefulness of garlic in dissolving clots. It therefore follows that daily garlic will be of help here, too.

An ancient remedy for piles practised by the apothecaries of old involved using a raw garlic clove as a suppository. It brings tears to my eyes to think about it, and I most certainly do not recommend it!

Chilblains

Circulatory problems are indicated if you suffer from chilblains. Applying garlic oil to the affected area, therefore, will help to reduce the local irritation. And, of course, eating garlic regularly will help to improve your circulation in general.

Male Impotence

At regular intervals throughout the garlic literature I have studied, the subject of impotence appears. For thousands of years, garlic has been hailed as a cure for male impotence. You may find this hard to believe, but if we consider how the penis becomes erect and how garlic works on the circulation, the connection may become clearer.

The penis contains an intricate pattern of numerous blood vessels, whose purpose is to hold as much blood as possible and thus maintain a firmly erect organ. One of the causes of male impotence is the inability of the penis to become erect because the vessels have started to become blocked with atheroma. Since garlic is effective at dissolving clots and opening up blood vessels, it might well do so on the blood vessels of the penis.

5

BALANCING YOUR DIET WITH GARLIC

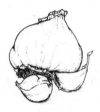

Although the main purpose of this book is to present the healthy effects of garlic consumption, these effects will be enhanced if you also take care about what you eat. The average man's body is composed of about 18 per cent protein, 14 per cent fat, 1.5 per cent carbohydrate and 62 per cent water, the remaining 4.5 per cent being minerals. To understand something of what the body requires to function efficiently, you need to know a little about protein and carbohydrate, as well as the benefits and problems of fats which I touched on earlier. Saturated, polyunsaturated and monounsaturated fats are discussed too glibly on television and in the press by a myriad of experts, each offering his or her suggestions on how to improve your diet.

Let's make one point clear at the outset. The word 'diet' to most people refers to weight loss. In this book I am referring to its other definition – the food we eat, its composition and its value to our health. Whatever the merits or demerits of the thousands of slimming diets on offer, my kind of diet is one which provides the necessary nutrition for healthy functioning of your body's organs, and plays a vital part in the proper development and function of your heart.

The Biochemistry of our Bodies

ESSENTIAL PROTEIN

For too many years we have read, seen and heard of the horrors of starvation in Africa and other parts of the world. Protein is essential in our diet and, whilst we can survive for some time with little or no carbohydrate or fat, a lack of protein rapidly causes death.

Good sources of protein include eggs, fish, meat, cheese, nuts and pulses. If you are a vegetarian, baked beans are an efficient source of protein. For good health, about 20 per cent of our daily energy requirement should come from protein.

Where Is Protein Manufactured?

Protein molecules are the largest in the body. They are constructed from strands of the twenty amino acids which are also present in the body. Protein is manufactured in many sites throughout the body, but the principal ones are the liver and muscles. The assembled amino acids which form the protein molecule are not uniform throughout the body, but have a composition peculiar to the site of the 'factory' that produces them.

As protein is used and broken down, a recycling system comes into play to synthesise more protein. If we relied on our diet to provide all the protein we need, the results would be disastrous. The amount of protein synthesised each day is about 300 grams, but the average Western diet provides only about 70 grams.

Protein as a Clotting Agent

Earlier, I described how fibrinogen was the basic protein involved in clot formation. Protein plays this essential role throughout the body. It is at work in the tissues of the arteries and veins, as well as in the skin and muscle.

Protein in Disease Protection

When we become infected with a virus or other organism, we normally produce antibodies which attack the invader. The main component of these antibodies is protein.

Back to LDL and HDL

Earlier, I explained how cholesterol is transported throughout the body in order to repair body cells and keep them healthy, and how excess cholesterol is removed to reduce the risk of clogging of the arteries. The two main components in this process are low-density lipoprotein (LDL) and high-density lipoprotein (HDL). Protein is the carrier for cholesterol.

CARBOHYDRATES FOR ENERGY

Our bodies run on energy like cars run on petrol. Energy is required at all levels of our daily existence – not just for obvious things like walking and running, but to enable every part of our bodies to function, right down to cellular level.

A normal, healthy body needs around 45 per cent of its daily energy intake to consist of carbohydrate which, after digestion, is absorbed into the body as glucose. The ideal amount for any individual depends on their age, sex, height, build and lifestyle. A manual worker, for instance, will need more carbohydrate than someone who works in an office; and a mother who is breast-feeding has higher requirements than a woman who is not. Everyone's carbohydrate needs decrease with age.

For a long time carbohydrates were regarded as the great fatteners, but this is not strictly speaking true. If you consume a lot of refined and processed foods – sweets, biscuits, cakes, soft drinks and so on – your body will produce a lot of energy very quickly. But unless you lead a very active life you will not use up all this energy, and your body will store it as fat. The healthy way to take carbohydrates is in the form of foods such as bread, pasta, cereals, potatoes, bananas, grapes and apples. These are metabolised more slowly by your body, and give you a kind of 'drip feed' of energy over several hours.

FATS

In the last twenty or thirty years, fats have been subjected to severe criticism by the medical profession in both the scientific press and the mass media. Fighting back, the margarine and butter manufacturers have spent millions on advertising campaigns in an attempt to persuade the public that their product – and their product only – is a healthy one. It is not surprising that some people have become confused and now regard all fat as harmful. Books have been written which advocate the removal of all fat from the diet – a dangerous attitude. I hope to set the record straight here, starting with a short description of the function of the various fats: saturated, unsaturated, monounsaturated and polyunsaturated.

Saturated Fats

The saturated fats consist of a group of fatty acids, of which lauric acid, myristic acid, palmitic and stearic acids are the commonest. In the British diet, with its emphasis on red meat and dairy products, palmitic acid is the kind most often encountered.

These fats are often referred to, understandably, as animal fats. But this leads people to believe that their only source of fat is in meat, milk, cheese and so on. This is a dangerous over-simplification. Some plant oils, for instance palm oil, contain these unhealthy saturated fats, while certain animal meats contain much safer unsaturated fats. This is particularly so for creatures which live in a cold environment. It's logical when you think about it. Saturated fats, such as butter or lard, are often solid or semi-solid when cold. Can you imagine a fish being able to swim about in near-Arctic waters if its body fat was saturated? It would be like a solid block of lard!

Cholesterol, Triglycerides and Saturated Fat

Without doubt, the saturated fats have more effect on the triglycerides and cholesterol than any other element in our diet. In countries where large amounts of saturated fats are consumed, the general level of blood cholesterol tends to be high, as does the incidence of heart disease.

Do All Saturated Fats Raise Cholesterol?

The answer to this question is that they do not – or, at any rate, that they do so to different degrees. Carefully controlled studies have shown that myristic acid raises cholesterol more than palmitic acid. What this means is that products containing butter fat, coconut oil and palm oil (all myristic acids) may raise your blood cholesterol to a greater degree than the fats in red meat.

This means we must be selective about the fat-containing foods that we eat. For most of us, a careful look at the fats in our diet and a general reduction in saturated fats is required. Our daily fat consumption should not produce more than 30 per cent of our energy requirement. Even then, most of this fat intake should consist of polyunsaturated and monounsaturated fats (see below, and pages 94-95 for foods which contain these).

Monounsaturated Fats

It is only recently that a real interest in the monounsaturated fats has emerged, with the evidence that people who live in Mediterranean countries have significantly less coronary heart disease than northern Europe and the USA. The reason for this is a number of differences in diet, including their consumption of olive oil. This oil contains monounsaturated fatty acids, as does rapeseed oil, which can now also be bought in the form of margarine.

Apart from olive oil, red wine and garlic may also have their part to play in protecting the inhabitants of Mediterranean countries from heart problems. Red wine is thought to contain antioxidants which, if you remember, catch free radicals. And the reduction in cholesterol produced by consuming olive oil is insignificant when compared to the effects of garlic on cholesterol. In addition, I am not aware of any significant changes in platelet stickiness in people eating olive oil, but I am in those eating garlic.

Polyunsaturated Fats

There are two main groups of polyunsaturated fats, called omega 6 and omega 3. The omega 6 fatty acids occur in plants such as maize, safflower and sunflower. Their main functions are as a source of energy and as components of the fats used in the body's structure. Because they are so important and cannot be manufactured in the liver, they are known as the essential fatty acids.

To show how essential omega 6 fatty acids are, we must go back to the 1930s when George and Mildred Burr, two Californian biochemists, were conducting experiments with the diet of rats. If their laboratory rats were deprived of all fats, they developed strange skin lesions and did not grow properly. The Burrs carefully added back into their diet, one by one, all the nutrients that were regarded as essential at that time. But there was no improvement. The Burrs labelled the elusive missing component 'vitamin F'. It was eventually discovered that vitamin F was linoleic acid, one of the omega 6 polyunsaturated acids. When it was added to the rats' diet, their skin problems cleared up and the animals developed normally.

Linoleic acid is taken up by the liver to form arachidonic acid, which is transported to the cells and tissues of the body. The purpose of arachidonic acid is to be converted, as required, into compounds known as prostaglandins. Among the vital functions prostaglandins perform are regulating blood clotting, childbirth contractions, and blood pressure. That is why it is called an essential fatty acid.

The Tale of Nurse B

During the many years in which I held a cholesterol clinic, it was not unusual for a doctor or practice nurse to sit in while I discussed blood test results with patients. On this particular day, Nurse B came along with one of her patients who had tried to lose weight and cholesterol for a considerable time, but without success. The patient said she had recently heard about a fat-free diet which was receiving a lot of publicity at the time. As I was explaining the dangers of such a diet, and using the research of George and Mildred Burr as an example, I saw the expression on Nurse B's face change and she began to look rather uncomfortable.

It transpired that Nurse B had recommended the fat-free diet, and was also using it herself. As I told my story, she began to realise why she had suddenly developed a skin problem. A month later, Nurse B told me her skin had returned to normal after she had started to include polyunsaturated fatty acids in her diet once more.

The omega 3 fatty acids exist in the most basic form of marine life, plankton. Fish feed on the plankton and themselves become rich in omega 3 fats. They are also found in the blubber of sea animals such as whales and seals. Because these fats stay fluid at such low temperatures, they enable these creatures and cold-water fish to keep mobile and function properly.

It has been suggested that this is why the Eskimos, who eat large quantities of fish rich in omega 3, do not suffer from heart attacks. Omega 3 fats reduce the blood triglycerides and, in the longer term, the LDL cholesterol. They also increase the HDL cholesterol and the bleeding time, and have a beneficial effect on platelets.

This group of fatty acids is responsible for normal growth, and research has demonstrated that one of them is essential for proper brain development. My earlier book *The Eskimo Diet* (see Further Reading on page 176) contains much more on the advantages of omega 3.

The Western Diet and its Faults

In Chapter 1 I wrote about the history of garlic and how it was mentioned in a number of herbal remedies in the Codex Ebers, an Egyptian medical papyrus of 1555 BC. The same manuscript includes the following passage: 'If thou examinest a man for ill-ness in his cardia, and he has pains in his arm, in his breast and in one side of his cardia ... then though shalt say thereof: it is due to something entering into the mouth, it is death that threat-ens him.'

'Cardia' refers to the chest in this astonishing, and probably earliest, reference to a heart attack. Even in those far-off days, it was realised that diet played an important part in the mainte-nance of good health and in particular to a healthy heart.

Let's now look at the types of food we typically eat, and see what we should be eating more of and what we should be eating less of. Remember, it is perfectly possible to eat healthily and enjoy your food, provided you follow one or two guidelines and use your common sense.

FIBRE

We hear a lot of experts extolling the virtues of fibre, which can indeed help many digestive and bowel conditions. So what is fibre? We have a bony skeleton to hold us together, and something similar applies to plants. Most vegetables, cereals and fruits have a distinctive shape and construction, and fibre is the material which forms the 'skeleton' of the plant.

It has been said that the reason people in the Third World suffer from fewer of the diseases that afflict us is their consumption of fibre. Black Africans, for instance, eat about four times as much fibre every day as we do: they do not have a problem with bowel cancer or irritable bowel syndrome, and constipation is rare. Fibre can also help to reduce cholesterol, and it is an important dietary aid to preventing some forms of cancer.

We need to increase the amount of fibre in our diet to about 35 grams daily; the current average in northern Europe and the USA is 14-18 grams. But don't overdo your fibre consumption – too much can produce a lot of gas and result in discomfort, and may even prevent essential nutrients being absorbed into the body.

Remember that not all fibre is useful. For instance, soluble fibres such as pectin from apples and oat gum from oat bran are excellent in the fight against high cholesterol. Wheat bran, however, is not effective in this connection because it is an insoluble fibre. The answer seems clear: an apple a day, together with vegetables and other fruits, can keep you regular while reducing your cholesterol. Eating fibre can also help to satisfy your appetite, and so aid weight loss.

Sources of Fibre

Apart from fruit and vegetables, already mentioned, there are various other good sources of fibre readily available on the supermarket shelves. Wholemeal bread is good, as are some of the breakfast cereals – check the packet for fibre levels. Potatoes are an excellent way of getting more fibre as well as taking in more of the right kind of carbohydrate for energy. For maximum benefit, bake them in their skins, and eat the skins, too.

Rice, particularly brown rice, is also fibre-rich. If you buy canned foods, the fibre, protein, carbohydrate and fat content will be printed on the label.

SATURATED FAT AND HOW TO CUT DOWN

I have already explained how saturated fats are not only responsible for high blood cholesterol levels, but also assist in the development of cancer. So it is in the best interests of us all to reduce consumption of all fat to 30 per cent or less of our dietary calories. I suspect that, if we were to reduce this figure to 25 per cent or less, the atheroma clogging our arteries would very gradually start to disappear. It is almost impossible to remove all the saturated fat from our diet. The most we can do is assess each food's saturated fat content and reject or reduce our intake of it accordingly.

Which Foods are High in Saturated Fats?

Beef, lamb and pork all contain fat, of which about 40-50 per cent is saturated. A good start is to cut off all the visible fat, but don't forget the 'hidden' fat between the lean fibres. This hidden fat is, however, greatly reduced in cooking.

Lard, suet and dripping are extremely high in saturated fats and should be avoided. Sausages, corned beef, bacon and hot dogs are also on the hit list and should only be eaten occasionally, as should liver, which has a high cholesterol content. (Liver, remember, is where cholesterol is manufactured.)

For many years eggs were considered to be very bad for your heart because of their cholesterol level, and many people suggested motting them altogether. Times change, and it is now thought that two or three eggs a week pose little or no threat to our health. But when calculating the number you are eating, you must allow for eggs used in cooking. For instance, a Yorkshire pudding for four will usually contain at least one egg.

Although fish is in general healthy – and some fish extremely good for you – there is one exception. Fish roe contains too much cholesterol, and should be avoided.

Another main source of saturated fats are dairy products. Full cream milk is high on the list, while skimmed milk has almost none. If you are like me and think that water tastes better than skimmed milk, use semi-skimmed instead. Cream, butter, cheeses and ice cream should also be eaten sparingly because of their high saturated fat content. Look for low-fat equivalents wherever possible.

When you buy vegetable oils for cooking, beware of palm oil and coconut oil which have an unacceptably high saturated fat content. Coconut also happens to be very rich in triglyceride. When serving any dish, unless it has a very low fat content in itself, try not to serve accompanying sauces or dips. In my view, these are just as responsible for our high saturated fat intake as the foods mentioned above.

Many people boast that they don't eat puddings and desserts because they are unhealthy and make them put on weight. What they don't say is that they often fill up with sweet biscuits, cheese and crackers, chocolate, or something similar. Cakes and biscuits taste as they do because they contain high levels of saturated fats. In the evening, when you go into the kitchen to make a cup of tea or to let the dog or cat out, don't eat the odd biscuit in the belief that, because it isn't very big, it can't do much harm. If you make this a habit, you will eat a lot of saturated fat. Think about the increasing risk of a heart attack – and be strong.

POLYUNSATURATES – GOOD FATS

Foods containing the polyunsaturated fats do not generally increase your cholesterol. In fact, many people regard them as a help in reducing cholesterol. Polyunsaturated fats occur in the seed oils such as sunflower and corn (maize), and in nuts. They contain the essential nutritional fat-soluble vitamins and, of course, the fatty acids that are vital for the proper development and functioning of humans. When you buy a margarine, low-fat spread or cooking oil, make sure the bottle or packet indicates that the contents are high in polyunsaturates. The table here is a useful guide for non-branded products.

Saturated fat content of fats and oils

grams of saturated
fat per 100g/3½ oz

Cooking fats

Solid beef fat (dripping)	59
Solid vegetable fat	26–50
Solid white cooking fat	47
Pork fat (lard)	38

Cooking oils

Coconut oil	85
Palm oil	49
Groundnut oil	19
Safflower oil	16
Soya oil	14
Grapeseed oil	14
Olive oil	13.4
Sunflower oil	13
Corn oil	11
Blended cooking oil (best quality)	7

Other Foods that Contain Polyunsaturates

Turkey and chicken do contain some saturated fat, but if the skin is removed most of this fat goes with it. Poultry contains polyunsaturated fat and is a wise choice – with the exception of duck and goose, which contain too much fat.

The fat content of fish varies greatly, but many of them, particularly the oily ones, contain omega 3 fatty acids (see page 90). These are most prevalent in cold-water fish such as salmon, mackerel, herring, sardine, anchovy, sea trout and tuna. So get into the habit of eating fish regularly to help protect your heart.

The recipes in Part 2 of this book contain several fish and garlic dishes. What could be better than to sit down to a delicious meal containing two of the most powerful and natural heart protectors available?

MONOUNSATURATED – MORE GOOD FATS

The best known of the oils rich in monounsaturated fats is, of course, olive oil which is used extensively in the mediterranean countries. Olive oil is one of the safer fats to include in our diet, and I have used it in several recipes in Part 2 of this book. In my opinion, it makes a valuable addition to many meals, particularly as a salad dressing. It should be used, where possible, in place of any of the other oils and fats.

BEWARE TRANS FATTY ACIDS

These fatty acids are produced when oils are hardened, as in the production of margarine. They are considered by many researchers to be even more likely to cause heart and artery problems than the saturated fats. Indeed, some doctors now recommend using a little butter as a spread rather than the conventional margarines. This seemed to be a very worrying development, until the margarine manufacturers tackled the problem by producing low-fat spreads with negligible amounts of trans fatty acids.

HOW HEALTHY IS A VEGETARIAN DIET?

Nowadays, a large number of people prefer not to eat meat for one reason or another. One of the questions often asked at my lectures concerns the possibility of vegetarians becoming anaemic, because they do not get the iron contained in red meat. Nothing could be further from the truth. Many vegetables contain sufficient iron for our daily needs – in fact, lentils have a higher content, weight for weigh, than meat. So continue to enjoy your vegetarian diet; it will most probably help to keep your blood cholesterol at a healthy level.

CONVENIENCE FOODS

Generally speaking, foods such as beefburgers, meat pies, fried fish, chips and cheeseburgers all contain a lot of fat. For every 100 grams of product, you will receive up to 30 grams of fat, a considerable proportion of which will be saturated. Think before buying convenience foods, and if you can't resist them, don't make a habit of it.

HOW SHOULD WE COOK OUR FOOD?

When you read the recipes you will find that very little frying is involved. It is acceptable to fry food in a little oil to seal in the juice (for instance, cubes of meat that are to go in a casserole), but to fry a full meal is asking for trouble. Fish should be grilled, baked or poached, and chips, although not forbidden, should only be eaten occasionally. When you do fry, use olive oil or one with a low saturated fat content (see table on page 94), and try to avoid butter, ghee (clarified butter), hard margarines and lard. Here is a useful checklist of healthy cooking and eating guidelines:

- Don't serve rich sauces with meat and poultry
- Liver and kidney are high in cholesterol, so eat only a little
- Sausages contain a lot of hidden fat, so eat them only occasionally
- Use semi-skinned or skimmed milk on and in your food
- Post-menopausal women should get plenty of calcium from milk and low-fat products to help prevent osteoporosis
- Examine labels on packaged food. Buy those that are low in saturated fats, but high in mono or polyunsaturated fats
- Avoid cakes, sweets, biscuits and chocolate because of their hidden fats
- Reduce your use of saturated fats and keep up the level of polyunsaturates
- Increase your use of monounsaturated fats
- Reduce your own and your family's fat consumption to 30 per cent of total daily calories
- Reduce salt and sugar consumption
- Eat more fibre
- Drink alcohol only in moderation – but don't forget the red wine, because it may help
- Use garlic liberally in cooking and take a capsule of garlic oil every day

How to Take Your Daily Garlic

CAPSULES

There are two ways of taking garlic: in your food, and in the form of capsules. Of the two, the latter is more important because fresh garlic alone will not provide you with enough of the active sulphur compounds.

There are about thirty different companies supplying garlic supplements in capsule or tablet form, some of which contain added vitamins or fish oil.

A garlic preparation which has had its effect on human patients adequately researched is Hofel's Cardiomax, garlic oil capsules, which I can recommend as the result of my research.

The suggested dose of Hofel's Cardiomax capsules is one a day which seems fine for most people but if you wish to significantly reduce your blood cholesterol levels, three capsules daily is more realistic. Three will give a daily dose of 12mg garlic oil. But please do not stop taking any prescribed medication without first consulting your doctor.

However, Hofel's garlic oil is encapsulated in gelatine and is unsuitable for vegans. If you are vegetarian I would suggest you try garlic tablets with parsley.

I also regard free radicals as a source of many health problems, so I take a capsule each of the antioxidants vitamin E, selenium and vitamin C. All the capsules mentioned here are available in health food shops.

FRESH GARLIC

It is easy enough to eat garlic in your food, and if you have never cooked with it before you should try some of the recipes in Part 2 – you may find you really enjoy its wonderful, tangy flavour. Most supermarkets and lots of greengrocers now sell garlic, so you should have no trouble obtaining it.

Dealing with Garlic Breath

A lot of people worry about smelling unpleasant after eating garlic. Chewing a little parsley or sucking a slice of lemon will help to remove the smell of garlic from your breath.

Part 2: Recipes

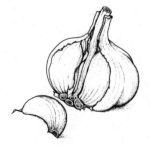

When you buy garlic, choose plump, firm bulbs which feel heavy in the hand. Pull the papery outer skin away to reveal the individual cloves. Remove as many as the recipe calls for, then skin them and cut off their hard bases. It is a matter of individual preference whether or not you use a garlic press to crush the skinned cloves – a sharp knife and a chopping board will do just as well.

Keep unused and partly used garlic bulbs in a cool, dry place – not the refrigerator, where they tend to go mouldy.

The recipes that follow are divided into sections, but there is, of course, no need to stick rigidly to these divisions. The ingredient quantities for a number of the dishes listed as snacks or starters, for instance, can easily be increased to make main courses. Likewise, vegetarians will find a number of non-meat recipes in the various sections. Just follow your instincts, get into the kitchen, use your garlic and enjoy good food and good health!

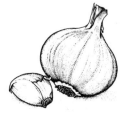

SOUPS, STARTERS AND SNACKS

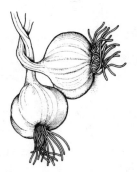

Thick Vegetable and Bean Soup
Serves 4-6

225g (8oz) haricot beans, soaked overnight in cold water
45ml (3 tablespoons) olive oil or sunflower oil
1 garlic clove, crushed
1 onion, chopped
2 sticks celery, sliced
3 carrots, sliced
450g (1lb) green cabbage, finely shredded
1 sprig each rosemary and thyme, tied together
15ml (1 tablespoon) tomato purée
salt and black pepper
30ml (2 tablespoons) chopped parsley
croûtons (see page 174)

Drain the beans, then place them in a large pan with 1.7 litres (3 pints) water. Bring to the boil and simmer, covered, for 2 hours or until tender.

Using a large, deep pan, heat the garlic, onion, celery and carrots gently in the oil. Stir frequently, until the vegetables are soft and have slightly browned. Add the cabbage and herbs, stir, and continue cooking for 4 minutes.

Drain the beans and add the liquid to the vegetables, together with the tomato purée and salt and pepper to taste. Bring the pan to the boil and simmer for 30 minutes. Then add the beans, together with more water if necessary, and simmer until the vegetables are tender. Remove the rosemary and thyme, and check the seasoning. Stir in the parsley, scatter the croûtons on top and serve immediately.

Lentil Soup
Serves 4

900ml (1½ pints) water
5ml (1 teaspoon) brewer's yeast extract
275g (10oz) lentils
1 large carrot, chopped
1 garlic clove, chopped or crushed
1 onion, chopped
15ml (1 tablespoon) tomato purée
300 ml (1½ pints) semi-skimmed milk
salt and pepper

Heat a little of the water in a small saucepan, add the yeast extract and stir until dissolved. Place the remaining water in a large pan, add the dissolved yeast extract and the lentils. Cover the pan, bring to the boil and leave for a few seconds. Then remove the pan from the heat and leave it to stand overnight.

Next day, bring the pan of lentils to the boil and add carrot, garlic, onion and tomato purée. Simmer, covered, for one hour. Blend the flour with a little of the milk to make a smooth paste, then stir into the remaining milk. Add this mixture to the pan, stirring all the time, add salt and pepper to taste, and simmer for 2 minutes until the soup has thickened.

Serve with toast.

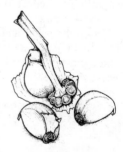

Minestrone
Serves 6

225g (8oz) haricot beans, soaked overnight in water
60ml (4 tablespoons) olive oil or rapeseed oil
2 garlic cloves, chopped or crushed
1 large onion, chopped
3–4 sticks celery, sliced
3 medium carrots, finely chopped
1 courgette, chopped
450g (1lb) tomatoes, skinned (see below), seeded and chopped
125g (4oz) green beans
125g (4oz) cabbage, shredded
1.7 litres (3 pints) vegetable stock from cubes
1 rasher lean back bacon, chopped into small pieces
75g (3oz) small pasta shapes or spaghetti broken into small pieces
8 tablespoons chopped parsley
salt and pepper
Parmesan cheese, grated

Cook the garlic and onion in the oil in a large pan until soft. Add the remaining vegetables, mix well, add the stock and bacon and bring to the boil. Simmer, covered, until the vegetables are almost tender. This should take about 40 minutes. Stir in the drained beans and the spaghetti or pasta and simmer for a further 15 minutes. Season to taste and serve sprinkled with Parmesan cheese.

Note: to skin tomatoes easily, drop them for about a minute into just-boiled water, then remove them with a slotted spoon and drop them into cold water. In another minute or so their skins should come off in your fingers, though you may need the point of a kitchen knife to start the process off.

Vegetarians can leave the bacon out of this recipe and make an equally delicious soup for a cold winter's day.

Summer Tomato Soup
Serves 4

450g (1lb) tomatoes, skinned (see page 109), seeded and chopped
100g (4oz) cucumber, peeled and chopped
1 garlic clove, chopped or crushed
small pinch cayenne
pinch salt
10ml (2 teaspoons) Worcestershire sauce
1 medium green pepper, cored, seeded and chopped
140ml (5oz) low-fat yoghurt

Place all the ingredients, except half the green pepper and the yoghurt, into an electric blender and work until smooth. Chill well. Stir in the remaining green pepper and yoghurt and garnish with chopped parsley.

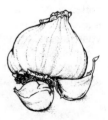

Cucumber Soup
Serves 4

500ml (1 pint) vegetable stock from a cube
1 cucumber, peeled and chopped
1 onion, chopped
2 garlic cloves, crushed or finely chopped
15ml (1 tablespoon) sunflower oil
15g (1oz) plain flour
100ml (4fl.oz) semi-skimmed milk
salt and pepper

Boil the stock and add the cucumber, onion and garlic. Cook until the onion softens, then briefly blend the mixture in an electric blender. Heat the oil in a large, deep pan, add the blended cucumber mixture and cook for 4–5 minutes, stirring continually. Blend the flour with a little of the milk to make a smooth paste, then stir in the remaining milk. Add the mixture to the pan and simmer for 2 minutes, stirring constantly, until the soup has thickened. Add salt and pepper to taste.

Serve with croûtons (see page 174).

Note: Meat or vegetable stock cubes are convenient, but fresh stock, if available, can be substituted in this or any other recipe. Just make sure that any fat is skimmed off the top before you use it.

Fish Chowder
Serves 4

450g (1lb) fresh cod fillets
30ml (2 tablespoons) olive oil
1 medium onion, finely chopped
I garlic clove, chopped
1 green pepper, cored and seeded
1 x 400g (14oz) can chopped tomatoes
10ml (2 teaspoons) tomato purée
225g (8oz) boiled potatoes, chopped
salt and black pepper

Cut the fish into small pieces. Heat the oil and cook the onion, garlic and green pepper until tender. Add all the other ingredients except the fish, and simmer for 15 minutes. Add the fish and cook for about 5 minutes until it flakes. Add salt and pepper to taste.

Serve with croûtons (see page 174) or toast.

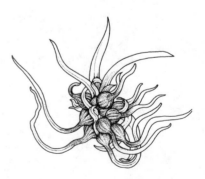

Shrimp and Mushroom Salad
Serves 4

100g (4oz) frozen shrimps, thawed
150g (5oz) fresh mushrooms
1 medium lettuce
parsley

Dressing:
1 garlic clove, finely chopped or crushed
½ teaspoon English mustard
salt and pepper
15ml (1 tablespoon) olive oil
30ml (2 tablespoons) wine vinegar

Slice the mushrooms and place them in a salad bowl with the shrimps. Combine all the dressing ingredients and add the mixture to the bowl. Toss thoroughly and serve on a bed of lettuce, garnished with parsley.

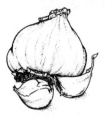

Scampi
Serves 4

450g (1lb) fresh jumbo shrimps
100g (4oz) polyunsaturated margarine
2 garlic cloves, crushed
15g (1 tablespoon) chopped frozen parsley
15ml (1 tablespoon) freshly squeezed lemon juice
½ teaspoon salt
pepper

Shell the shrimps and wash them well in cold water. Remove the sand vein by making a deep cut down the back of the shrimp, at the same time opening up the shrimp in butterfly fashion. Place the margarine, garlic, parsley, lemon juice and salt in a shallow, microwave-safe dish. Microwave on high for 2 minutes, then stir in the shrimps until they are fully coated. Add a shake of pepper and continue cooking on top of the stove, uncovered, for 4–5 minutes, stirring occasionally. Take care not to cook for too long or the shrimps will become tough.

Serve with fresh bread and/or salad.

Note: This is a partly microwave recipe for occasions when you don't have a lot of time, but it could easily be adapted to conventional cooking.

Tuna Pâté
Serves 3–4

1 x 213g (7oz) tin tuna in brine
salt and pepper
15g (½ oz) low-fat spread
1 garlic clove, roughly chopped
15g (½ oz) plain flour
300ml (½ pint) semi-skimmed milk
1 x 11g sachet gelatine
150ml (¼ pint) low-fat yoghurt

Place the tuna in a sieve and wash out the excess brine with cold water. Chop it finely and add salt and pepper to taste.

Heat the low-fat spread in a small pan together with the garlic. After a minute, remove the garlic and discard. Add the flour and heat, stirring, for 2 minutes. Remove the pan from the heat and gradually stir in the milk. Bring to the boil and simmer, stirring, for 1–2 minutes. Mix the sauce with the tuna. Make up the gelatine according to the instructions on the packet, and stir into the tuna mixture. Let it cool slightly, then mix in the yoghurt and lemon juice and pour the pâté into a serving dish.

Chill in the refrigerator for 2 hours, garnish with tomato or cucumber slices if you like, and serve with toast.

Kipper Pâté
Serves 4

1 packet kipper fillets
75g (3oz) low-fat spread
50g (2oz) small mushrooms, sliced
1 garlic clove, cut in two
zest and juice of ½ lemon
pinch nutmeg
freshly ground black pepper
100ml (4fl.oz) low-fat yoghurt

Pre-heat the oven to 190°C (375°F/gas mark 5). Place the kippers in a dish, dot them with a little of the low-fat spread, and bake for 15 minutes.

Drain the juices from the cooked kippers into a small pan. Add the mushrooms and garlic and cook on a high setting for 2 minutes, shaking all the time. Discard the garlic.

Place the cooked kipper fillets, juices, the rest of the low-fat spread, the lemon juice and zest in a blender. Add the nutmeg and pepper to taste, and liquidise until smooth. Stir the yoghurt into the pâté and chill for 2 hours.

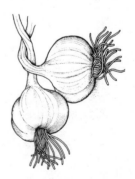

Fish Kebabs
Serves 4

250g (9oz) fresh salmon fillet
250g (9oz) fresh cod fillet
1 garlic clove, chopped or crushed
45ml (3 tablespoons) sunflower oil
45ml (3 tablespoons) soy sauce
30ml (2 tablespoons) medium or dry sherry
15ml (1 tablespoon) demerara sugar
½ tablespoon orange zest

Cut the fish into cubes large enough to fit on to skewers, and place the cubes in a deep dish. Mix together all the other ingredients and pour over the fish. Marinate at room temperature for 1 hour.

Grease the 4 skewers and thread the fish pieces on to them, alternating the cod and salmon. Barbecue or grill on one side, then brush on some of the leftover marinade and turn the skewers to cook the other side. Cook until the fish flakes easily but is still firm.

Adeje Omelette
Serves 4

3 medium Spanish onions, chopped
2 garlic cloves, chopped or crushed
30ml (2 tablespoons) olive oil
5–6 eggs
pinch salt and black pepper

Fry the onions and garlic in the oil in an omelette pan. Beat the eggs with the salt and pepper and stir them into the onion and garlic mixture. Cook until the underside is just browning. Sprinkle the top with a little grated hard cheese and place under grill until top surface is no longer runny.

Serve immediately with fresh bread and/or mixed salad.

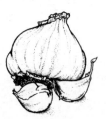

Stuffed Tomatoes
Serves 4

4 large tomatoes
15ml (1 tablespoon) olive oil
1 onion, chopped
1 garlic clove, finely chopped
50g (2oz) mushrooms
50g (2oz) grated Cheddar cheese
50g (2oz) breadcrumbs
salt and freshly ground black pepper
50g (2oz) prawns

Pre-heat the oven to 190°C (375°F/gas mark 5). Slice the tops off the tomatoes and remove the seeds and centres. Put the empty tomato shells to one side, and sieve the seeds and centres to make a pulp.

Heat the oil and fry the onion, garlic and mushrooms until tender. Add the grated cheese, sieved tomato pulp, breadcrumbs and salt and pepper to taste. Mix well, add the prawns and fill the tomato shells with the mixture. Bake for 10 minutes.

Garnish with sprigs of parsley and serve with toast.

MAIN MEALS: POULTRY

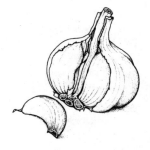

Chicken Risotto
Serves 4

30ml (2 tablespoons) olive oil
1 medium onion, sliced
1 garlic clove, cut in two
900ml (1½ pints) chicken stock from a cube
175g (6oz) rice, washed and drained
300g (11oz) cooked chicken, chopped
salt and pepper

Heat the oil in a deep pan. Fry the onion and garlic, taking care not to let the onion brown. Remove the garlic after 1 minute and discard.

Add the chicken stock and bring to the boil, then add the rice. Place a lid on the pan and simmer for about 20 minutes, giving it an occasional, very gentle stir. The dish is cooked when the rice has absorbed most of the stock. Add the chicken and season to taste.

Serve on its own, or with green salad.

Note: some rice is specially quick-cooking. Check the instructions on the packet so that you don't over-cook the risotto.

Chicken Casserole
Serves 4

15ml (1 tablespoon) vegetable oil
2 medium carrots, sliced
1 medium onion, chopped
2 garlic cloves, finely chopped or crushed
1 sprig thyme
1 bay leaf
450ml (¾ pint) chicken stock from a cube
4 chicken joints, skin removed
salt and pepper
225g (8oz) button mushrooms

Pre-heat the oven to 170°C (325°F/gas mark 3). Heat the oil in a pan and add the carrot, onion, garlic, thyme and bay leaf. Cook, stirring often, until the vegetables are just tender. Transfer them to a casserole dish and add the stock and chicken joints. Cook in the oven for 45 minutes, then add the seasoning and mushrooms. Cook for a further 15 minutes.

Serve with new potatoes and salad.

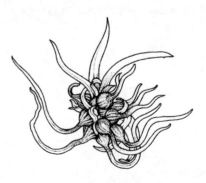

Chicken Espanol
Serves 4

30ml (2 tablespoons) sunflower oil
4 chicken joints, skinned
1 medium onion, sliced
2 garlic cloves, finely chopped or crushed
45ml (3 tablespoons) dry or medium sherry
1 chicken stock cube
110ml (¼ pint) water
3 large tomatoes, skinned (see page 109), seeded and chopped
2 teaspoons tomato purée
1 teaspoon arrowroot
chopped parsley

Heat the oil in a deep frying pan that has a lid, then add the chicken, onion and garlic. Add the sherry, stock cube and pre-measured water. Continue to cook until the stock cube has dissolved. Add the tomatoes and tomato purée and simmer for 20 minutes. Pre-heat the oven to 180°C (350°F/gas mark 4).

Remove the chicken and place in a casserole dish. Sieve the juices left in the pan. Mix the arrowroot with a little water and boil for 2–3 minutes until clear. Stir into the sieved juices and pour this sauce over the chicken in the casserole dish. Cook for 1 hour.

Coq au Vin
Serves 4

30ml (2 tablespoons) sunflower oil
4 chicken joints, skinned
4 very small onions
1 garlic clove, finely chopped or crushed
30ml (1 tablespoon) plain flour
450ml (1 pint) chicken stock from a cube
225ml (8 fl.oz) red wine
225g (8oz) mushrooms, left whole if small or sliced if large
1 teaspoon sugar
1 sachet bouquet garni
salt and black pepper

Pre-heat the oven to 180°C (350°F/gas mark 4). Heat the oil in a frying pan and fry the chicken pieces until just golden. Remove the chicken and put on one side in a warm place. Add the whole onions and garlic to the pan and fry until the onions are tender. Add the flour, mix well with the juices in the pan, and cook for about 2 minutes. Slowly stir in the stock and red wine and cook until the sauce has thickened. Add the mushrooms, sugar and bouquet garni. Season to taste.

Transfer the sauce and chicken pieces to a casserole dish with lid. Cook for 45 minutes or until tender. Remove the bouquet garni.

Serve with Basmati rice or mashed potato.

Garlic Chicken in Wine
Serves 4

4 chicken breasts, skinned
1 garlic clove, finely sliced
30ml (2 tablespoons) olive oil
300ml (½ pint) medium or dry white wine
½ teaspoon salt
75g (6 oz) mushrooms, sliced
25g (1 oz) cornflour
45ml (3 tablespoons) water

With a sharp knife, make small incisions in the chicken pieces and push slices of garlic into them. Heat the oil in a frying pan and fry the chicken gently until just browned all over. Add the wine, salt and mushrooms and simmer for about 30 minutes or until the chicken is tender. Remove the chicken and keep in a warm place. Mix the cornflour to a creamy consistency with the measured water, add to the mixture in the pan and stir continuously until the sauce has thickened. Put the chicken pieces back into the pan and briefly reheat.

MAIN MEALS: FISH

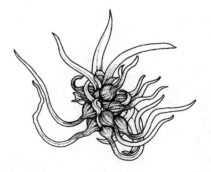

Stuffed Mackerel
Serves 4

4 small to medium fresh mackerel, cleaned, with
heads and backbone removed
3 tablespoons chopped onion
50g (2oz) fresh breadcrumbs
1 teaspoon finely grated orange zest
1 eating apple, peeled, cored and grated
10ml (2 teaspoons) lemon juice
2 teaspoons chopped fresh chives
1 garlic clove, chopped
salt and freshly ground black pepper
60ml (4 tablespoons) orange juice

Pre-heat the oven to 180°C (350°F/gas mark 4). Wash and dry the fish. Mix together the onion, breadcrumbs, orange zest, apple, lemon juice, chives, garlic, and season with salt and pepper. Divide the stuffing mixture into four and fill the cavity in each fish. Roll the fish up, secure each with a cocktail stick and place them in a greased ovenproof dish. Pour the orange juice over the fish and cover with foil. Bake for about 20 minutes or until the fish is cooked through.

Garnish with slices of orange and watercress and serve hot or cold.

Stuffed Herrings
Serves 4

225g (8oz) freshly prepared wholemeal breadcrumbs
2 tablespoons chopped parsley
1 garlic clove, very finely chopped
1 medium onion, finely chopped
1 medium cooking apple, peeled and finely chopped
1 teaspoon mixed herbs, fresh or dried
salt and pepper
1 egg
4 herrings, cleaned

Pre-heat the oven to 180°C (350°F/gas mark 4). Thoroughly mix the breadcrumbs, parsley, garlic, onion, apple, herbs and salt and pepper to taste. Beat the egg and stir well into the stuffing mixture. Add a little water if the mixture does not bind well. Divide the stuffing into four and fill the cavities in the herrings. Transfer the fish to a greased oven-proof dish, cover with foil and bake for about 20 minutes until tender.

Serve cold, garnished with slices of lemon and accompanied by a salad.

Pickled Herrings
Serves 4

8 medium herring fillets
zest and juice of 1 orange
1 teaspoon wild garlic vinegar
salt
1 garlic clove, thinly sliced
a few peppercorns
4 bay leaves
1 medium onion, sliced

Pre-heat the oven to 190°C (375°F/gas mark 5). Roll up the herrings, skin outside, and secure them with cocktail sticks. Grease a small ovenproof dish with a little sunflower oil and add the herrings. Pour the orange juice and wild garlic vinegar over the herrings, and sprinkle the zest, a little salt, the garlic and the peppercorns on top. Put the bay leaves in the dish and arrange the sliced onion over the herrings. Pour over just enough water to cover the herrings. Bake, covered, for 30 minutes.

When cold, remove the fish from the liquid and serve with fresh crusty bread.

Fried Monkfish Pieces
Serves 4

350g (12oz) monkfish tail, skinned and
cut into cubes about 2.5cm (1 inch) square
a little plain flour
60ml (4 tablespoons) olive oil
1 teaspoon mixed herbs, fresh or dried
2 cloves garlic, finely chopped or crushed
salt and black pepper
15ml (1 tablespoon) freshly squeezed lemon juice

Coat the monkfish in plain flour and fry in the oil in a small frying pan.
Mix in the herbs, garlic, and salt and pepper to taste. Fry for just a few
minutes, until the fish is golden. Pour lemon juice on top.
   Serve with new potatoes and lemon wedges.

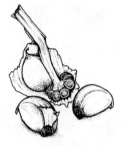

Grilled Salmon
Serves 4

1 garlic clove, roughly chopped
30ml (2 tablespoons) sunflower oil
4 salmon steaks 2.5cm (1 inch) thick
a little lemon juice
salt and black pepper

Fry the garlic in the oil over a gentle heat for 3 minutes. Reserve the oil but discard the garlic. Wash the salmon steaks and dry them on kitchen paper. Place the fish on oiled baking foil on the grill tray, squeeze a little lemon juice on top, season lightly and brush some of the garlic-flavoured oil on to the fish. Grill for about 5 minutes, then turn the fish over and repeat the process for the other side.

Garnish with lemon slices and parsley sprigs.

Saucy Salmon Steaks
Serves 4

4 x 175–225g (6–8oz) salmon steaks
50g (2oz) polyunsaturated margarine
1 garlic clove, finely chopped or crushed
a few peppercorns
45ml (3 tablespoons) fresh lemon juice
½ teaspoon chopped fresh dill
¼ teaspoon sugar
salt

Wash the salmon steaks, pat them dry on kitchen paper and put them in a microwave-safe dish. Place the margarine, garlic, peppercorns, lemon juice, dill, sugar and salt to taste in a jug and microwave on high for about 1–1½ minutes, stirring half-way through. The margarine should by now be melted. Brush some of this sauce over the salmon steaks and microwave on medium for 8–10 minutes, turning the salmon half-way through the cooking cycle. Leave for 5 minutes. Reheat the remaining sauce, if necessary, and pour it over the fish.

Garnish with lemon slices and parsley, and serve with new potatoes and mangetout.

Note: this dish can easily be adapted for conventional cooking if you don't have a microwave.

Spanish Cod
Serves 4

1 onion, finely chopped
1 garlic clove, finely chopped or crushed
1 tablespoon olive oil
½ green pepper, cored, seeded and sliced
4 tomatoes, skinned (see page 109) and sliced
4 x 150g (5oz) cod fillets, skinned
25g (1oz) plain flour
10 stuffed olives
150ml (¼ pint) white wine

Cook the onion and garlic in a little of the olive oil until just tender, then add the green pepper and tomatoes and cook gently for a further 2–3 minutes. Remove the pan from the heat, but keep it warm. Heat the remaining oil in a separate pan. Coat the cod fillets with flour and fry until cooked through, turning once. Add the olives and white wine to the onion and tomato mixture and reheat. Pour the sauce over the fish.

Serve with green salad and new potatoes.

Cod with Yoghurt
Serves 4

1 small can sild or sardines in oil
1 large onion, chopped
1 garlic clove, finely chopped or crushed
45ml (3 tablespoons) olive oil
4 medium tomatoes, skinned (see page 109)
chopped fresh parsley
salt and black pepper
4 x 150g (5oz) cod fillets
90ml (6 tablespoons) yoghurt

Remove the sild from the oil and mash it up (discarding the oil). Place it with the onions and garlic in a frying pan and cook in the olive oil until the onions are golden. Quarter the tomatoes, add to the pan and cook gently for a further 2–3 minutes. Add the parsley, and salt and pepper to taste, then put the mixture into a large, shallow, lightly greased flameproof dish. Pre-heat the grill on its highest setting. Place the cod fillets on the mixture and grill for 5–6 minutes. Then add the yoghurt, reduce the grill temperature slightly, and cook for a further 7 minutes or until the fish is cooked through.

Cod Salad
Serves 4

4 x 175g (6oz) cod steaks
2 garlic cloves, finely chopped or crushed
1 small onion, finely chopped
30ml (2 tablespoons) olive oil
45ml (3 tablespoons) medium or dry white wine
3 tablespoons chopped parsley
salt and pepper

Place the fish in a shallow dish. Mix all the other ingredients and pour over the fish. Leave to marinate for 3–3½ hours. Then remove from the marinade, steam for 15 minutes and leave to cool.

Serve with a mixed salad and cooled baby new potatoes.

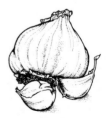

Italian-style Fish
Serves 4

4 x 150g (5oz) cod or haddock fillets
a little plain flour
30ml (2 tablespoons) vegetable oil, plus a little extra for frying
1 medium onion, sliced
1 garlic clove, finely chopped or crushed
60ml (4 tablespoons) dry white wine
15ml (1 tablespoon) wild garlic vinegar
salt and pepper
2–3 sage leaves, crumbled
1 teaspoon sugar

Wash the fish and cut it into strips about 2.5cm (1 inch) wide. Coat them in flour, and fry in a little oil until golden brown. Drain.

Make the marinade by first heating the measured oil in a pan and gently frying the onion and garlic for 6–7 minutes or until slightly coloured. Then add the wine, garlic vinegar, salt and pepper to taste, sage and sugar, and simmer for 2 minutes. Pour the mixture over the fish and allow to cool before serving.

Tuna Tagliatelle
Serves 4

15ml (1 tablespoon) olive oil
1 medium onion, finely chopped
1 garlic clove, finely chopped or crushed
30ml (2 tablespoons) red wine
1 x 400g (14oz) can chopped tomatoes
15ml (1 tablespoon) tomato purée
1–2 courgettes, sliced
1 teaspoon wild garlic vinegar
1 x 400g (14oz) can tuna in brine, drained, rinsed in water and flaked
2 teaspoons chopped basil
black pepper
400g (14oz) dried tagliatelle

Heat the olive oil in a frying pan and cook the onion and garlic until the onion is tender. Add the red wine, tomatoes, tomato purée, courgettes and wild garlic vinegar. Reduce the heat and cook for 4–5 minutes. Add the tuna, basil and pepper and heat through. Remove from the heat and keep hot.

Put the tagliatelle in a large pan of boiling water and cook according to the instructions on the packet. Drain, place the tagliatelle on to individual plates and pour the sauce on top.

Salade Niçoise
Serves 4

1 lettuce
225g (8oz) green beans, boiled and cut small
225g (8oz) new potatoes, cooked and diced
6 spring onions, sliced
1 red pepper, cored, seeded and sliced
1 x 200g (7oz) can tuna in brine, drained, washed and flaked
50g (2oz) anchovy fillets, drained and cut into strips
2 tablespoons capers
60ml (4 tablespoons) French dressing

To finish:
4 hard-boiled eggs (tulip-cut, if possible)
4 medium tomatoes, cut into wedges
a few black olives, according to taste

Arrange the lettuce leaves on individual plates or in a large salad bowl. In a separate bowl, mix the beans, potato, spring onions, red pepper, tuna, anchovies and capers. Pour the dressing on top, toss lightly and spoon the mixture on to the lettuce. Place the egg, tomatoes and olives on top.

Serve with hot, crusty bread rolls.

Note: you can use ready-made French dressing, or prepare your own by pouring 3 tablespoons olive oil and 1 tablespoon vinegar in a screw-top jar and shaking vigorously. Add salt and pepper to taste. (For Salade Niçoise, however, you probably won't need any extra salt because there is plenty in the anchovies).

Shrimp Curry
Serves 6

15ml (1 tablespoon) olive oil or sunflower oil
1 onion, chopped
2 garlic cloves, finely chopped or crushed
1 large eating apple, peeled, cored and chopped
165g (6oz) shrimps
225ml (8fl.oz) water
45ml (3 tablespoons) curry paste
110g (4oz) frozen peas, thawed
25g (1oz) plain flour
a little lemon juice

Heat the oil in a pan, add the onion, garlic and apple and fry until almost tender. Remove the vegetables from the pan and add the shrimps. Fry for about 1 minute. Return the vegetables to the pan and add the measured water and the curry paste. Bring to the boil, reduce to a simmer and add the peas. Mix the flour with a little water to make a creamy consistency and add to the pan, stirring all the time. When the mixture thickens, simmer, covered, for 10 minutes.

Squeeze lemon juice over the curry and serve with boiled Basmati rice.

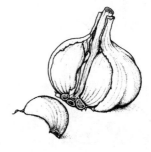

Garlic Prawns with Rice
Serves 4

225g (8oz) Basmati rice
30ml (2 tablespoons) olive oil
150g (5oz) prawns, thawed if frozen
2 garlic cloves, peeled and crushed
100g (4oz) frozen peas, thawed
black pepper
2 large eggs
soy sauce

Wash the rice and boil in salted water, according to the instructions on the packet, until tender. Heat the olive oil in a wok or deep frying pan and gently fry the prawns, garlic and peas for about 5 minutes. Season to taste with the pepper. Remove from the frying pan and keep warm. Place the cooked rice in the frying pan, add the eggs and fry for about 5 minutes, stirring well. Return the prawns, garlic and peas to the pan and mix them thoroughly with the rice. Add soy sauce to taste, and serve garnished with lemon slices if desired.

Squid in Tomato Sauce
Serves 4

15ml (1 tablespoon) olive oil
450g (1lb) squid, cut into strips
1 large onion, chopped
2 garlic cloves, finely chopped or crushed
1 x 225g (8oz) can chopped tomatoes, drained
1 bay leaf
large pinch dried marjoram
1 teaspoon wild garlic vinegar
225ml (8fl.oz) red wine
black pepper

Heat the oil in a deep frying pan and fry the squid until golden. Add the onion and garlic and fry for a few minutes more, until the onion is tender. Add the tomatoes, bay leaf and marjoram, and cook for a further 5 minutes. Stir in the wild garlic vinegar and red wine and simmer, covered, for about an hour, until the squid is tender. Season to taste.

Serve with Basmati rice.

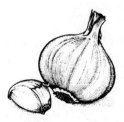

Garlic Mussels
Serves 4

30ml (2 tablespoons) sunflower oil
1 small onion, chopped
1 garlic clove, finely chopped or crushed
1 x 200g (7oz) can chopped tomatoes
½ teaspoon mixed herbs
900g (2lb) mussels in their shells
225ml (8 fl.oz) dry white wine
1 teaspoon wild garlic vinegar
black pepper

Heat the oil in a frying pan and cook the onion and garlic over a gentle heat until the onion is tender. Add the tomatoes and mixed herbs and cook, covered, for 10 minutes.

Wash the mussels and throw away any with shells that are open. Pour the wine into a large pan, add the mussels, bring to the boil and simmer until the shells open. Throw away any mussels with shells that remain shut. Remove the beard and half the shell from the good mussels, leaving the mussels on the other half-shell.

Strain the wine in which the mussels were boiled, add the wild garlic vinegar, then add to the onion and tomato mixture. Season with pepper and reheat gently for 2 minutes.

Serves with fresh crusty bread or garlic bread (see page 173).

Paella
Serves 4

30ml (2 tablespoons) olive oil
4 tomatoes, skinned (see page 109)
1 medium onion, chopped
1–2 garlic cloves, finely chopped or crushed
100g (4oz) Basmati or long-grain rice
small pinch saffron
600ml (1 pint) chicken stock from a cube
salt and pepper
225g (8oz) halibut
225g (8oz) fresh haddock or cod
225g (8oz) mussels (see page 146), boiled and with beard and top shell
removed
1 green pepper
1 teaspoon wild garlic vinegar
175g (6oz) prawns, fresh or frozen (thawed)

Heat the oil in a large, deep frying pan. Quarter the tomatoes and fry
them with the onion and garlic until the onion is tender. Add the rice
and stir. Add the saffron to the chicken stock and pour into the pan.
Season with salt and pepper to taste and simmer for 7–10 minutes. Add
the fish, the mussels, the green pepper and the garlic vinegar. Cook
gently until the rice has swollen and is soft. Add the prawns and cook
only until they are heated through, which takes about 2 minutes. Pour
the Paella on to a large warmed serving dish and garnish with parsley.

MAIN MEALS: MEAT

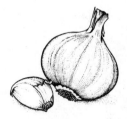

Italian-style Meatballs
Serves 4

2 slices white bread, crusts removed
300ml (½ pint) semi-skimmed milk
450g (1lb) leg of beef
50g (2oz) fresh parsley
1–2 cloves garlic
40g (1½ oz) Parmesan cheese, grated
2 eggs, beaten
pinch grated nutmeg
salt and pepper
olive oil for frying

Soak the bread in the milk for a few minutes. Mince the meat with the parsley, garlic and soaked bread. Add the cheese, eggs, nutmeg and seasoning to taste, and mix well. With the help of a little flour, roll the mixture into balls about 4cm (1½ inches) in diameter. Fry in hot olive oil for 3–4 minutes, until cooked through. Then transfer to a larger pan if necessary, and simmer, covered, in tomato sauce (see page 172) for 20 minutes.

Serve with boiled rice or pasta.

Spanish Meat Loaf
Serves 4

2 rashers lean back bacon with fat removed
225g (8oz) lean minced beef, cooked and with the fat skimmed off
2 slices wholemeal bread, made into breadcrumbs
300ml (½ pint) semi-skimmed milk
1 garlic clove, finely chopped or crushed
1 teaspoon mixed herbs
pinch paprika
½ teaspoon salt
pinch celery salt
150ml (¼ pint) water
1 x 200g (7oz) can chopped tomatoes
50g (2oz) long-grain rice, boiled in salted water

Pre-heat the oven to 180°C (350°F/gas mark 4). Mince the bacon and add it to the minced beef. Soak the breadcrumbs in the milk and add to the meat mixture. Add the crushed garlic, herbs, paprika and salt. Add celery salt to taste, and stir in the measured water, tomatoes and rice. Grease a bread tin with a little olive or sunflower oil and add the meat loaf mixture. Cook for 35–40 minutes.

Serve hot with a green salad and potatoes.

Stewed Steak with Onions
Serves 4

700g (1½ lb) lean stewing or braising steak, cut into 2.5cm (1 inch)
cubes
a little plain flour
25ml (1½ tablespoons) sunflower oil
2 large onions, sliced
2 garlic cloves, finely chopped or crushed
1 beef stock cube
150ml (5fl.oz) water
1 bay leaf
salt and pepper

Pre-heat the oven to 180°C (350°F/gas mark 4). Coat the beef with flour, then fry quickly in hot oil until browned on all sides. Place in an ovenproof casserole and add the onions and garlic. Dissolve the beef cube in the measured water, then add to the casserole along with the bay leaf. Cover, and cook for 2 hours.

Serve straight from the cooking dish, accompanied by mashed potato and vegetables.

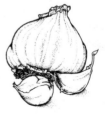

Spaghetti Bolognese
Serves 4

30ml (2 tablespoons) olive oil
1 medium onion, chopped
1 garlic clove, finely chopped or crushed
450g (1lb) lean minced beef, cooked and with the fat skimmed off
1 x 225g (8oz) can chopped tomatoes
50g (2oz) small mushrooms, sliced
15ml (1 tablespoon) tomato purée
1 teaspoon Italian mixed herbs
1 teaspoon wild garlic vinegar
beef stock from a cube
black pepper
225g (8oz) spaghetti

Heat the oil in a frying pan and cook the onion and garlic until the onion is tender. Add the minced meat and stir. Continue cooking until the meat browns, then add the tomatoes, mushrooms, tomato purée, herbs, garlic vinegar, stock and pepper to taste. Boil for 1½–2 minutes, then simmer for a further 25 minutes, adding more stock if needed.

Bring a large pan of water to the boil and add the spaghetti, cooking according to the instructions on the packet. Strain, tip on to a large, hot serving dish, pour the sauce on top and serve accompanied by a bowl of grated Parmesan cheese.

Corned Beef Hash
Serves 4

30ml (2 tablespoons) olive oil
225g (8oz) corned beef, chopped
1 small onion, chopped
1 garlic clove, chopped
6 medium potatoes, boiled
110g (4oz) frozen mixed vegetables, thawed
45ml (3 tablespoons) beef stock from a cube
ground black pepper

Heat the oil in a frying pan and fry the meat, onion and garlic for 2–3 minutes. Add the potatoes, vegetables and the stock, with pepper to taste, and heat through until just brown, stirring constantly. Turn out into a hot dish and serve.

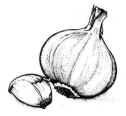

Country Casserole
Serve 4

45ml (3 tablespoons) olive oil
1 large onion, sliced
1 garlic clove, finely chopped or crushed
1 cooking apple, peeled, cored and chopped
450g (1lb) white cabbage, shredded
1 green pepper, seeded and chopped
450g (1lb) lean stewing or braising steak, cubed
a little plain flour
225g (8oz) canned tomatoes without liquid
100ml (4fl.oz) red wine
100ml (4fl.oz) beef stock
2 chicken breasts, cubed
salt and black pepper

Pre-heat the oven to 180°C (350°F/gas mark 4). Heat the oil and fry the onion and garlic until the onion is just tender. Add the apple, cabbage and green pepper, and continue cooking, stirring all the time, for about 2 minutes. Place in a large casserole with a lid.

Coat the beef in flour and fry quickly until sealed and golden brown. Transfer the beef to the casserole, along with the tomatoes, red wine and beef stock. Cover the casserole and cook for one hour, then add the chicken pieces and cook for a further hour. Add salt and pepper to taste.

Serve with boiled potatoes or a crusty loaf.

Hungarian Cabbage Parcels
Serves 4

1 medium onion, chopped
2 garlic cloves, finely chopped or crushed
75g (3oz) long-grain rice, boiled and drained
225g (8oz) very lean rump steak, chopped or minced
225g (8oz) very lean pork, chopped or minced
8 large green cabbage leaves, washed
15ml (1 tablespoon) wine vinegar
2 large tomatoes, skinned (see page 109) and chopped
salt and pepper

Combine the onion, garlic, rice, steak and pork. Place the cabbage leaves in hot water and soak them until they are soft enough to form envelopes around the filling. Tie each little parcel with thread, or secure with cocktail sticks, so that the filling cannot escape. Place the vinegar and tomatoes in a pan with a very little water, bring to the boil, add the cabbage parcels and simmer gently until the cabbage has turned brown. Season to taste.

Serve with mashed potato.

Stuffed Gammon with Glazed Onions
Serves 4

1 small packet sage and onion stuffing
juice of ½ lemon
2 x 225g (8oz) lean gammon steaks with all visible fat removed
16 very small onions
1 tablespoon polyunsaturated margarine
1 teaspoon sugar

Pre-heat the oven to 200°C (400°F/gas mark 6). Make up the stuffing according to the instructions on the packet, adding the lemon juice. Spread a layer of stuffing on each gammon steak and roll them up. Grease an ovenproof dish with a little oil to prevent sticking, place the two stuffed gammon rolls in it, cover with greaseproof paper and bake for 30 minutes.

Put the onions in a pan with some cold water and bring to the boil. Strain, add the margarine and sugar, and cook gently for about 20 minutes, shaking constantly, until onions are tender.

To serve, cut each stuffed gammon steak in two and accompany with the onions and boiled potatoes.

Note: if you have the time, this recipe would be even nicer with a home-made stuffing.

Stuffed Peppers
Serves 4

225g (8oz) low-fat sausage meat
1 medium onion, chopped
4 slices bread, made into breadcrumbs
½ clove garlic, finely chopped or crushed
60ml (4 tablespoons) olive oil or sunflower oil
2 sticks celery, chopped
1 teaspoon marjoram
1 tablespoon fresh, chopped parsley
salt and pepper
1 lemon
4 red, green or yellow peppers

Pre-heat the oven to 190°C (375°F/gas mark 5). Combine the sausage meat, onion, breadcrumbs and garlic and fry in hot oil until light brown and just tender. Add the celery, marjoram, parsley, and salt and pepper to taste. Squeeze the juice of a lemon over the top and mix well.

Cut the tops off the peppers and remove the core and seeds. Then simmer the peppers in salted water for 4–5 minutes. Drain, and fill with the sausage meat mixture. Place the stuffed peppers in a greased baking tin and cook for 25 minutes.

Serve immediately with tomato sauce (see page 172) and mashed potato or boiled rice.

Garlic Roasted Lamb
Serves 4–6, depending on the size of the joint

leg of lamb
2–3 cloves of garlic, thinly sliced
rosemary sprigs
black pepper
45ml (3 tablespoons) sunflower oil

Pre-heat the oven to 190°C (375°F/gas mark 5). Make small incisions all over the surface of the joint and carefully insert a slice of garlic into each. Also place the rosemary sprigs into a number of the cuts. Sprinkle with pepper.

Place half the oil in a roasting tin and add the lamb. Pour the rest of the oil over the joint and cook for about 30 minutes per 450g (1lb), plus an extra 30 minutes. To test, push a fork into the meat: if the juices run clear, the joint is cooked. Leave the meat to 'relax' in a warm place for 10–15 minutes. This makes it easier to carve and more tender to eat.

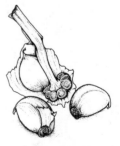

Lamb Casserole
Serves 4

4 lamb loin chops
a little plain flour
30ml (2 tablespoons) sunflower oil
1 large onion, ½ sliced, ½ chopped
1 garlic clove, chopped
4 medium tomatoes, skinned (see page 109) and chopped
600ml (1 pint) meat stock from a cube
1 teaspoon wild garlic vinegar (see page 109)
salt and pepper

Pre-heat the oven to 180°C (350°F/gas mark 4). Coat the chops in the flour. Heat the oil in a pan and fry the chops until slightly browned. Remove the chops to a plate and fry the onions and garlic (you may find it easier to use two frying pans at this stage, since the chopped onions are supposed to be kept separate from the sliced onions). Put the chopped onions in a casserole dish, place the chops on top and then cover with the sliced onions. Add the tomatoes, stock and garlic vinegar. Season with salt and pepper to taste and cook in the oven for 1 hour.

Serve with boiled or mashed potatoes, mint sauce and peas.

VEGETARIAN DISHES

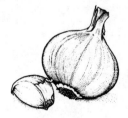

Stir-fried Mushrooms
Serves 4

1 garlic clove, cut in half
small piece root ginger (about 15mm/½ inch long)
60ml (4 tablespoons) olive oil
1 onion, finely sliced
1 small leek, finely sliced
175g (10oz) small mushrooms
pinch of salt
1 teaspoon soy sauce

Place the garlic pieces and ginger in a wok or frying pan with the oil and cook, stirring occasionally, for 1–1½ minutes. Remove the ginger and garlic (or you can leave the garlic in the pan, if you prefer), add the onion and leek and fry for another 1–2 minutes. Add the mushrooms and fry for another 2 minutes. Sprinkle over the salt, followed by the soy sauce.

Serve with noodles or Basmati rice.

Vegetable Casserole au Gratin
Serves 4

2 medium onions, sliced
1 small turnip or swede, chopped
450g (1lb) carrots, sliced
225g (8oz) frozen mixed vegetables
450g (1lb) potatoes
40g (1½ oz) polyunsaturated margarine
1 garlic clove, roughly chopped or sliced
40g (1½ oz) plain flour
450ml (¾ pint) semi-skimmed milk
salt and pepper
175g (6oz) low-fat Cheddar cheese, grated

Pre-heat the oven to 180°C (350°F/gas mark 4). Boil the onions for 3–4 minutes until they are just starting to soften, then add the turnip and carrots. Cook until tender, then add the mixed vegetables, and cook fur a further 2 minutes. Strain, retaining the liquid.

Boil the potatoes in salted water and, when cool enough to handle, cut into thick slices.

Heat the margarine with the garlic in a deep pan. Then remove the garlic, mix in the flour and cook, stirring, for 2 minutes. Remove from the heat and slowly stir in the milk, together with 150ml (¼ pint) of the vegetable liquid. Put the pan back on the heat and cook slowly, stirring, until the mixture thickens. Add salt and pepper to taste, and half the cheese.

Mix this sauce thoroughly into the vegetables, then grease a casserole dish and pour the mixture in. Cover with the sliced potatoes followed by the remainder of the cheese. Place in the oven and cook for 25 minutes.

Serve hot, accompanied by a salad if desired.

Grilled Potato Slices with Onion and Tomato
Serves 4

2 large onions, thinly sliced
4 large potatoes, thickly sliced
25g (1oz) polyunsaturated margarine
25g (1oz) plain flour
225ml (8oz) semi-skimmed milk
salt and pepper
100g (4oz) low-fat Cheddar cheese, grated
4 medium tomatoes, sliced

Boil the onions and potatoes in salted water until tender, then strain and place in a shallow ovenproof dish. Pre-heat the grill.

In a separate pan, melt the margarine, add the flour and cook, stirring, for 2 minutes. Slowly add the milk, stirring continually. Cook the mixture until it thickens, add seasoning to taste, then pour the sauce over the onions and potatoes. Cover with grated cheese and tomato slices and place under the grill until the cheese is brown and bubbling.

ACCOMPANIMENTS TO OTHER DISHES

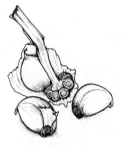

Savoury Rice
Serves 4

225g (8oz) Basmati rice
30ml (2 tablespoons) sunflower oil
1 garlic clove, finely chopped
1 medium onion, finely chopped
1 large tomato, skinned (see page 109) and seeded
1 teaspoon wild garlic vinegar
1 large egg, beaten
10ml (2 teaspoons) soy sauce
salt and pepper

Wash the rice, drain and boil in sufficient salted water to cover it by about 12mm (½ inch). Stir occasionally, and boil for 10 minutes or so, until all the water has been absorbed and the rice is swollen and tender. Fluff up the rice with a fork, place on one side and keep warm.

Heat the oil and fry the garlic and onion until the onion is tender. Chop the tomato, add to the pan along with the wild garlic vinegar, and cook for a few minutes. Add the rice, then stir in the egg and soy sauce. Cook for 1–2 minutes and season to taste.

Tomato Sauce

25g (1oz) polyunsaturated margarine
15ml (1 tablespoon) olive oil
1 medium onion, chopped
2 garlic cloves, finely chopped or crushed
450g (1lb) ripe tomatoes, skinned (see page 109) and chopped
large pinch sugar
salt and pepper
1 teaspoon each of dried oregano, dried
thyme, chopped fresh parsley and chopped fresh basil

Heat the margarine and oil in a pan and gently fry the onion and garlic until softened. Add the tomatoes to the pan with the sugar, and salt and pepper to taste. Bring to the boil, then simmer for about 12 minutes until most of the liquid has evaporated. Finally, stir in the herbs. Leave for 10 minutes to allow the flavours to amalgamate.

This sauce is equally delicious served hot or cold.

Garlic Bread
sufficient for 2 slices

15g (½ oz) polyunsaturated margarine
1 garlic clove, crushed or garlic purée
2 slices of bread

Pre-heat the grill. Mix the margarine thoroughly with the crushed garlic or about 10cm (4 inches) of garlic purée from a tube. Divide this mixture equally and spread on the 2 slices of bread. Place under the hot grill until toasted, and serve very hot.

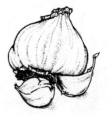

Croûtons

olive oil, for frying
1 clove garlic, chopped
4 slices wholemeal bread

Heat the olive oil and garlic in a pan. Dice the bread into very small cubes and add to the hot oil. Cook until crisp and golden, then drain on kitchen paper.

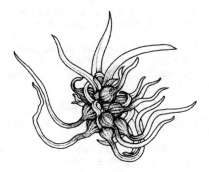

SOURCE REFERENCES

BARRIE, S.A., Wright, J.V. and Pizzorno, J.E., 'Effects of garlic oil on platelet aggregation, serum lipids and blood pressure in humans', *Journal of Orthomolecular Medicine* 1987; 2: 15–21.

DEBOER, L.W.V. and Folts, J.D., 'Garlic extract prevents acute platelet thrombus formation in stenosed canine coronary arteries', *American Heart Journal* 1989; 117: 973–975

GUNN, J., Gillott, T., Collings, K., Taylor, T., Tsikaderis, D., Vassilopoulus, A. and Saynor, R., 'A prospective, open label, dose ranging study of the effects of garlic in mixed hyperlipidaemia', *American Heart Association* 1994; 67th Scientific Session, November.

HARENBURG, J., Giese, C. and Zimmerman, R., 'Effect of dried garlic on blood coagulation, fibrinolysis, platelet aggregation and serum cholesterol levels in patients with hyperlipoproteinaemia', *Atherosclerosis* 1988; 74: 247–249.

JAIN, R.C. and Konar, D.B., 'Effect of garlic oil in experimental cholesterol atherosclerosis', *Atherosclerosis* 1978; 29: 125–129.

JUNG, F., Kieswetter, H., Mroweitz, C., Pindur, G., Heiden, M., Miyashita, C. et al., 'Akutwrikung eines zusammengesetzen Knoblauchprapartes auf die Fließfähigkeit des Blutes', *Zeitschrift für Phytotherapie* 1989; 10: 87–89.

KLEIJNEN, J., Knipschild, P. and Ter Riet, G., 'Garlic, onions and cardiovascular risk factors. A review of the evidence from human experiments with emphasis on commercially available preparations', *British Journal of Clinical Pharmacology* 1989; 28: 533–544.

LAU, B.H., Lam, F. and Wang-Cheng, R., 'Effect of an odour modified garlic preparation on blood lipids', *Nutrition Research* 1987, 7: 139–149.

MAKHEJA, A.N. and Bailey, J.M., 'Antiplatelet constituents of garlic and onion', *Agents Actions* 1990; 29: 360–363.

MAKHEJA, A.N., Vanderhoek, J.Y. and Bailey, J.M., 'Inhibition of platelet aggregation and thromboxane synthesis by onion and garlic', *Lancet* 1979; i: 781.

MAYEUX, P.R., Agrawal, K.C., Tou, J.-S.H., King, B.T., et al., 'The pharmacological effects of allicin, a constituent of garlic oil', *Agents Actions* 1988; 25: 182–190.

NISHINO, H. et al., 'Anti-tumour promoting activity of garlic extracts', *Oncology* 1989; 46: 277–280.

SUMIYOSHI, H. and Wargovich, M.J., 'Garlic (Allium sativum): A review of its relationship to cancer', *Asia Pacific* 1989; 4: 133–140.

WARGOVICH, M. J. et al., 'Chemoprevention of n-nitrosomethylbenzylamine-induced oesophageal cancer in rats by the naturally occurring thioether diallyl sulfide', *Cancer Research* 1988; 46: 277–280.

WOLF, S., Reim, M., and Jung, F., 'Effect of garlic on conjunctival vessels: a randomised, placebo-controlled, double-blind trial', *British Journal of Clinical Practice* 1990; 44 (symp. suppl. 69): 36–39.

YAN, X., Wang, Z, and Barlow, P., 'Quantitative determination and profiling of total sulphur compounds in garlic health products using a simple GC procedure', *Food Chemistry* 1992; 47: 289–294.

YOU, W.C. et al., 'Allium vegetables and reduced risk of stomach cancer', *Journal of the National Cancer Institute* 1989; 81: 162–164.

FURTHER READING

FULDER, Stephen, *Garlic, the Life-blood of Good Health*, Thorsons, Wellingborough, 1989.

GIBNEY, Michael J., *Nutrition, Diet and Health*, Cambridge University Press, Cambridge, 1986.

ROSER, David, *Garlic for Health*, Martin Books, Cambridge, 1990.

SAYNOR, Reg and Ryan, Frank, *The Eskimo Diet*, Ebury Press, 1990.

USEFUL ADDRESSES

For information on garlic research:

David Roser
Garlic Research Bureau
PO Box 40
Bury St Edmunds
Suffolk
IP31 2SS

Supplies of garlic seed cloves:

For supplies of seed cloves and garlic paraphernalia from the UK's largest importers of garlic please write to:

Brookerpaks Ltd.,
Breach Lane,
Newington,
Kent.
ME9 7PR

For information on garlic oil in capsules and on vitamins:

Seven Seas Ltd
Hedon Road
Marfleet
Hull
HU9 5NJ

For details of suppliers of wild garlic vinegar and similar products:

Les Fines Herbes
8 St Mary's Hill
Stamford
Lincolnshire
PE9 2DP

INDEX

abscesses 5, 10
accompaniments to main meals 169–74
acne 77–8
Adam 14
Adeje omelette 118
adrenaline 33–4
age 45
ailments, everyday 75–82
alcohol 35, 44–5
allicin 16–17, 18
anchovies 142
antibacterial properties 10, 13, 63–4
antibiotic properties 9, 61
antioxidants 70, 71–2
aphrodisiac properties 8
apples
    cooking 132, 156
    eating 131, 143
arteries 5
arthritis 80
aspirin 53–5
Atherosclerosis 53
athlete's foot 78

bacon, back 152
Baghurst, Dr - 47
Barany, Dr - 66
Barlow, Dr Philip 16
Barrie, Dr S.A. 58
Bartley, Walter 28
beans
    green 109, 142
    haricot 107, 109
beef
    corned 155
    leg 151
    minced 152, 154
Beeton, Mrs Isabella 13
Belman, Dr - 66
Bible 7
biochemistry 84–90
Black Death 12–13
Block, Dr - 66
blood 8, 21–59
blood pressure 55–6, 58–9
boils 9–10, 77
Bordia, Professor - 30, 48, 53
botany 15–19
bread 151, 173, 174

bread crumbs 119, 131, 132, 152, 159
breath 11–12, 99
Britain 10–11, 13
British Medical Journal 32
bronchitis 8
bubonic plague 12–13
Burr, George 88–9
Burr, Mildred 88–9

cabbages 107, 109
    green 157
    white 156
Caesar, Julius 10
cancers 65–9
capers 142
capillaries 50–1
capsules of garlic oil 97, 98
carbohydrates 85–6
cardiovascular diseases 32
carrots 107, 108, 109, 124, 166
casseroles
    chicken 124
    country 156
    lamb 161
    vegetable 166
Castelli, Dr W. 28
celery 107, 109, 159
cheese, Cheddar 119, 166, 167
chemistry 15–19
Cheops 4
chicken 123–7
chicken casserole 124
chicken espanol 125
chicken risotto 123
chilblains 81
China 6
chives 15
cholesterol 5, 22–31, 87, 89, 93
chowder 112
circulation of blood 3–4, 37–43, 51–2
cod 112, 117, 137–40, 147
cod salad 139
cod with yoghurt 138
Codex Ebers 5, 90
colds 75–6
colic 11
Columella 9
contraception 36
cooking methods 23, 96–7

coq au vin 126
corned beef hash 155
coronary thrombosis 23, 32, 46–8
coughs 76
country casserole 156
courgettes 109, 141
croûtons 173
cucumber soup 111
cucumbers 110, 111
culinary properties 4, 6, 13
Culpeper, Thomas 3
curry, shrimp 143

diabetes 73–4
diarrhoea 80
diet
    balanced 83–99
    western 21–2
Dioscorides 10
dressings 13
dysentery 13

earache 76–7
Eden, Garden of 14
eggs 118, 132, 142, 144, 151, 171
Egypt, Ancient 4–5, 7
Eskimos 31–2
essential fatty acids 88–9
essential oil 18
Europe 8, 12–13
European Heart Journal 32
everyday ailments, remedies 75–82

family planning clinics 36
fats 33–4, 86–90
Fenwick, Dr G.R. 63
fibre 91–2
fibrinogen 48
fibrolytic activity 52–3
First World War 13
fish 112, 117, 129–47
fish chowder 112
fish kebabs 117
fish oil 53–5
flatulence 11
flu 75–6
Food, Science and Nutrition 63
France 8, 13
free radicals 70–1, 98
fried monkfish pieces 134
fungal infections 64

Gabon 13
Galen 9

gammon steaks 158
gangrene 9, 13, 63
Garden of Eden 14
garlic bread 172
garlic chicken in wine 127
garlic mussels 146
garlic prawns with rice 144
Garlic Research Bureau 16
garlic roasted lamb 160
general practitioners (GPs) 36
ginger, root 165
Giza, Egypt 4
grave goods 4
Great Plague 12–13
Great Smokies Medical Center, USA 58
Greece, Ancient 8–9
grilled potato slices with onion and tomato 167
grilled salmon 135
growing garlic 15, 64
Gupta, Dr - 52

haddock 140, 147
haemostasis 46–7
halibut 147
Hanley, Dr A.B. 63
Harrington, Sir John 12
heart 19, 37–40
    disease 3–4, 23–30, 32–5, 40–3
    free radicals 70–1, 73, 98
Henry IV, King of France 12
Herculaneum, Italy 9
herrings 132, 133
high blood pressure 55–6
high-density lipoproteins (HDL) 25–6, 28–9, 31,
    34–5, 85
Hippocrates 8
history 3–20
Homer 8
honey 77
Horie, Dr T. 72
Hungarian cabbage parcels 157
hypertension 56–7

Iliad 8
impotence, male 81
India 3–4
indigestion 80
infections, fungal 64
insect bites 4
insulin 74
Israelites 7
Italian-style fish 140
Italian-style meatballs 151
Italy 5

Jain, Dr - 29, 53
Jang, Dr - 67
Japan 18–19
Journal of the National Cancer Institute 67
Julius Caesar 10

kebabs, fish 117
Kiesewetter, Dr H. 52
kipper pâté 116
Knasmulle, Dr - 69

labile hypertension 56–7
lamb
    leg 160
    loin 161
lamb casserole 161
leeks 15, 165
lentil soup 108
lettuce 113, 142
Lin, DR X.Y. 68
longevity 6, 7
Lonicerus 11
low-density lipoproteins (LDL) 26–8, 29, 31, 72, 85
Lui, Dr J.Z. 68
lung diseases 11

mackerel 131
magical properties 14
main meals
    fish 129–47
    meat 149–61
    poultry 121–8
    vegetarian 163–7
Marcus Aurelius, Emperor 9
margarine 95–6
meat, main meals 149–61
meat loaf, Spanish 152
meatballs, Italian-style 151
methyl allyl trisulphide (MATS) 18–19
Middle Ages 11–12
Milner, Dr J.A. 68
minerals 15–16
minestrone 109
monkfish 134
monounsaturated fats 88, 95
mosquitoes 5, 79
mucus 9
mushrooms 116, 119, 126–7, 154
    button 124
    salad 113
    stir-fried 165
mussels 146

n-nitroso compounds (NOCs) 68
Nero, Emperor 9
non-pathogens 62–4
nuts 71

oil
    essential 18
    fish 53–5
omelettes 118
oranges 133

paella 147
Paracelsus 11
parasites 79
Pasteur, Louis 63
pathogens 62–4
Patsch, - 33
peas, frozen 143, 144
peppers
    green 110, 112, 137, 147, 156
    red 142, 159
Phoenicians 7–8
Phytotherapy 72
pickled herrings 133
piles 80
plague 12–13
Planta Medica 72
platelets 46–7, 53
pneumonia 8
polyunsaturated fats 88–90, 94–5
pork 157
potatoes 142, 155, 166, 167
poultry 121–8
prawns 119, 144, 147
proteins 84–5
    see also high-density lipoproteins; low-density lipoproteins
pyramids 4–5

radiation 68–9
red blood cells 50–2
remedies, everyday ailments 75–82
research programmes 28–31, 35, 58–9, 66–9, 72
respiratory properties 8, 11
Reuter, Dr H.D. 72
rice 123
    Basmati 144, 147, 171
    long-grain 147, 152, 157
risotto, chicken 123
Romans, Ancient 9–11
Roser, David 16

sage and onion stuffing mix 158
salad Niçoise 142

salads 139, 142
salmon 117, 135, 136
salt 57
Satan 14
saturated fats 86–7, 92–3
sauce, tomato 172
saucy salmon steaks 136
sausage meat 159
savoury rice 170
scampi 114
Schweitzer, Albert 13
selenium 16, 72
sexual stamina 8
Shakespeare, William 11
shallots 15
Sheffield University 28, 30, 35
shopping 103
shrimp curry 143
shrimp and mushroom salad 113
shrimps 113, 114, 143
Silk Road 6
Sinclair, Dr Hugh 31
sinusitis 76
smoking 41, 43–4
snacks 112–19
sore throats 76
soups 105–12
spaghetti bolognese 154
Spain 8
Spanish cod 137
Spanish meat loaf 152
spots 77
sprains 79–80
spring onions 142
squid in tomato sauce 145
stamina, sexual 8
starters 105–19
steak
    rump 157
    stewing 153, 156
Stensvold, Dr - 32
stewed steak with onions 153
stir-fried mushrooms 165
stress 56
stuffed gammon with glazed onions 158
stuffed herrings 132
stuffed mackerel 131
stuffed peppers 159
stuffed tomatoes 119
sulphides 16–17
Sumiyoshi, Dr - 66
swedes 166

tagliatelle 141

Terracotta Army 6
throats, sore 76
tomato sauce 171
tomato soup 110
tomatoes 142, 147, 161
    canned 112, 141, 145–6, 152, 154, 156
    large 119, 125, 157
    medium 161, 167
    skinned 109, 137, 138
trade 6, 7–8
trans fatty acids 95–6
triglycerides 5, 31–5, 50, 74, 87, 93
tumours 5
tuna 115, 141, 142
tuna pâté 115
tuna tagliatelle 141
turnips 166
Tutankhamun, Pharaoh 4

vampires 14
varicose veins 80
vegetable and bean soup 107
vegetable casserole au gratin 166
vegetable oil 23
vegetables, frozen 155, 166
vegetarian diet 96, 103, 163–7
veruccas 78
very low-density lipoprotein (VLDL) 27, 31
Vesuvius, Mount 9
vinegar
    wild garlic 133, 140–1, 145–7, 154, 161, 171
    wine 157
viscosity, blood 49, 51
vitamins 71–2
Vyas, Dr - 29

Wargovitch, Dr M.J. 66, 67
warts 78
Weisenberger, Dr - 47
wine
    red 88, 126, 141, 145, 156
    white 127, 137, 139, 140, 146
World Health Organisation (WHO) 30
worms 5, 11, 79

yeast extract 108
yeast infections 64
yoghurt 110, 115, 116, 138
You, Dr W.C. 67